KETO DIET for WOMEN AFTER 50

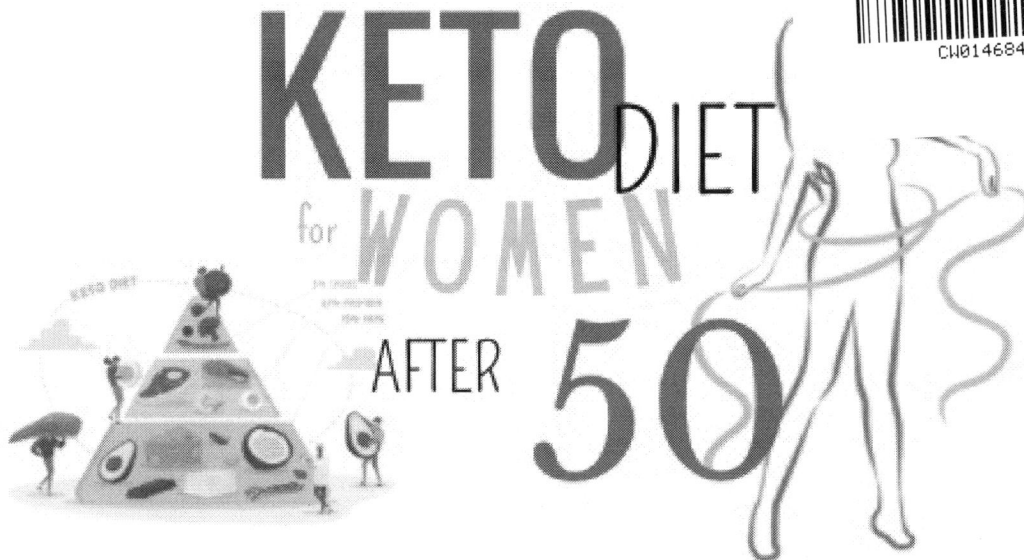

Complete Beginners Guide to
Fast Lose Weight and Shape Your Body!
300+ Easy, Tasty, Healthy & Low-carb Diet Recipes!
Regain Confidence & Balance Hormones!
+4week Meal Plan

BY

Eleanor Fields, Ph.D.

TABLE OF CONTENT

INTRODUCTION

THIS BOOK WANTS TO GUIDE YOU to quickly make a lifestyle change like millions of people have successfully made by eating healthy, natural, and delicious foods can help you feel and look exceptionally great! The Keto diet will provide your body with constant energy throughout your day, benefiting your mental and physical health. Indeed, by understanding the very basics of your body and dieting, you will reach your success without starving yourself, eating bland, without strictly counting calories, or go through various induction phases as for the classic diets, which cannot become a lifestyle.

The key to the success of the most effective diets is reducing foods rich in carbohydrates. Scientific studies in dietetics proved that making a low-carb diet and maintaining the same daily calories lose more weight than eating low-fat meals and reducing calories. Moreover, lowering the carbohydrates intake has shown an essential improvement in health indicators such as triglyceride, blood sugar, insulin levels, and more. Indeed, from a biochemical point of view, when you eat macromolecules as carbs, your digestive enzymes break them down into monomers (glucose), which is nothing but simple sugar. The produced glucose quickly and significantly raises your blood sugar levels; at this point, your body produces insulin to reduce this spike in blood sugar concentration. After many of these cycles, your body will need to make more insulin to achieve the same results. What does this mean? It means that you can quickly become insulin resistant, which leads to turning into a prediabetic person, develop a metabolic syndrome, and, eventually, type 2 diabetes mellitus (T2DM). According to researchers, T2DM is one of the most widespread metabolic diseases. Nowadays, enormous challenges in the diagnosis, prevention, and treatment of this disease are poses given the alarming rise in T2DM prevalence worldwide especially exploding in both low-income countries and adolescents/young adults, as well as the severe impact it has on longevity and quality of life (Izzo et al., 2021). Besides, more than 1 in 3 adults in the United States have prediabetes, and nearly 1 in 10 has type 2 diabetes. Furthermore, the number of obese adults has enormously spiked from 15 percent to 35 percent of all adults ages 20 to 74 in the last decade.

Food Pyramid Guide, which placed carbs into the base and a most extensive section of the pyramid, recommended that you eat many fruits (full of fructose, i.e., sugars) a day.

But there is some news for you: Do you know that your body can use your fats to convert glycerol into glucose? This process happens in your liver, and it is called gluconeogenesis!

You will now think that saturated and monounsaturated fats cause heart disease, cholesterol problems, and many other issues. In the last decades, multiple studies and meta-studies (the analysis of other studies' results) comprising millions of people showed that eating saturated and monounsaturated fats have no effects on heart disease risks even in the long-term. Indeed, there are both essential fatty acids and amino acids (monomers of protein). Carbohydrates and protein produce both 4 calories per gram and, on the other hand, fats generate more than double the amount of energy (about 9 calories), thus considered the most efficient form. When the introduced carbs are very low, and you eat lots of protein and fat, your body starts to convert free-fats and protein and the fat you have stored, into ketone bodies, or ketones, for energy by a metabolic process called ketosis. That's the key process of the ketogenic diet underpinnings.

Thanks to this book, you will succeed with the ketogenic diet by easy-to-cook meals achieving weight loss and long-term success.

Reference: Izzo A, et al. Nutrients. 2021. PMID: 33435310 Review.

CHAPTER 1: THE SCIENCE BEHIND THE KETO DIET

Let's start with the name of this diet: "keto" diet. The term "keto" refers to a metabolic state known as "ketogenic," which consists of a ketosis phase that starts in the body when carbohydrate intake is suddenly reduced and replaced with healthy fats. This diet is useful for losing stored fat in your body, resulting in your body's exceptionally productive shape and getting ripped.

The first step of the diet consists of a drastic reduction of carbohydrates consumption, which will help the body enter the ketosis metabolic state; during this state, the body will burn fat deposits rather than store glucose in glycogen form. Like the Mediterranean one, many diets suggest carbohydrates-based food intake (pasta, bread, etc.); when this daily macromolecule requirement is exceeded, the liver then converts it into glycogen. The body produces insulin to move the glucose in the bloodstream, transporting it through the body and the brain. But what is this glucose? It is sugar. And what sugar do? As said, when it reaches the brain affects your attention and concentration. Glucose is the body's primary energy source body, which will always use glucose over fats to produce the necessary energy.

The focus of the ketogenic diet is on using fat as a source of energy rather than glucose. When the body enters the ketosis state, it starts burning fat deposits, metabolizing them in ketones; this process will bring you to lose weight and improve your health. In fact, your "bad fat" (saturated) will shrink, helping your blood circulation, reducing the risk of heart attack, strokes, but also will reduce the sugar in your body, avoiding the onset of metabolic diseases such as diabetes.

Do you know that there are several types of ketogenic diet? No? Don't worry, let's see them together:

THE STANDARD KETOGENIC DIET (SKD)

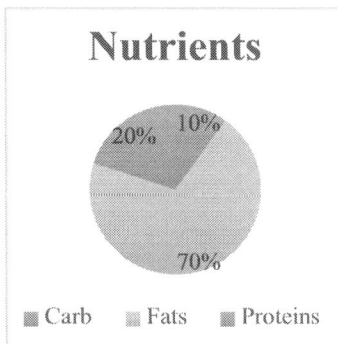

Nutrients

10%

20%

70%

■ Carb ■ Fats ■ Proteins

SKD consists of assuming a meager daily amount of carb, a high portion of fats, and moderate protein.

As shown in the pie chart, you should assume 70% of fats, 20% of protein, and 10% of carbs per day. It means that a person should eat 20-45 g of carbohydrates, 40-65 g of proteins without setting any limit for fats since it is the primary nutrient for this diet.

Now someone could think, why should I eat fats when I want to lose weight? This is because this diet uses fats as the primary source to produce energy by activating the ketogenic metabolic pathway.

The SKD is a suitable type of keto diet for those who want to lose weight and, at the same time, lower their sugar level in the blood and improve heart health.

CYCLICAL KETOGENIC DIET (CKD)

CKD diet's primary focus is on making 5 Ketogenic days and two high-carb days, and this cycle is repeated. This diet is also known as carb backloading. It is often intended for athletes because the diet allows their bodies to recover the glycogen lost due to workouts or intense sporting activities.

THE WELL FORMULATED KETOGENIC DIET

As the name suggests, this diet has its fats, carbohydrates, and proteins well-formulated to meet the standards of a Ketogenic diet. This diet is also similar to the SKD, which means that it creates room for your body to undergo Ketosis effectively.

THE MCT KETOGENIC DIET

We talk about MCT Ketogenic Diet when the Standard Ketogenic Diet refers to medium-chain triglycerides (MCTs). In this keto diet, coconut oil is substituting olive oil since it has high MCTs levels. MCTs allow your body to consume carbohydrates and proteins, maintaining the metabolism under ketosis. This process has been reported to help, and in some cases, treat epilepsy. But why are MCTs so efficient for the keto diet? Because MCTs are providing more ketones per gram in fat.

On the contrary, the long-chain triglycerides lower the ketones production, which is more common in the average dietary fats. However, this keto diet can provide some drawbacks like diarrhea and stomachache if the MCTs are consumed alone. So, what can I do to avoid drawbacks? Well, the solution is preparing the meal with the right balance of MCTs and "typical" fats. This diet is suitable for an athlete or for those who have some metabolic problem related to grain derivates' consumption.

THE CALORIE RESTRICTED KETOGENIC DIET

This keto diet is an SKD but with daily restricted calories. Researchers have already proven the efficacy of the ketogenic diet regardless of calorie consumption restriction. The base concept is that by consuming fats rich in calories, you will have the sensation of eating more, thus avoiding the typical over-eating.

After this overview regarding the different types of ketogenic diets, we can say that the Standard and the High-Protein Ketogenic diets are the most studied and recommended for health issues. However, for those who are practicing sports, like bodybuilding, the Targeted and Cyclical Ketogenic diets are the best ones to gain a good result; we should say that these two diets are for advanced people who want to upgrade to the next level compared to SKD.

Before starting any of these diets, visit and consult your local physician to understand which one is more suitable for you.

TARGETED KETOGENIC DIET (TKD)

TKD diet's primary focus is on the additional assumption of carbohydrates during the workout sessions only. The diet concept is very close to that of SKD, except when the carbs must be assumed (workout sessions). When you are exercising, the base concept is that the body will effectively and efficiently process carbohydrates consumed before or during a workout session. This is because the muscle needs and demands more energy when subjected to a higher physical effort; carbohydrates are polymers made by a chain of monomers (sugars), which are rapidly processed since the body is in a state of energy demand.

Briefly, this diet is a hybrid between the Standard Ketogenic Diet and the Clinical Ketogenic Diet, allowing little carbs consumption only when you are going to exercise.

HIGH-PROTEIN KETOGENIC DIET

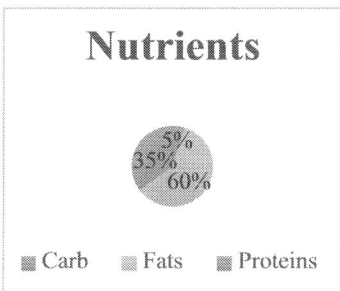

Nutrients

5%
35%
60%

■ Carb ■ Fats ■ Proteins

As suggested by its name, this Keto diet requires a higher daily percentage of protein assumption compared to the Standard Ketogenic Diet. This diet consists of intake of 35% of proteins (+15% concerning SKD), 60% of fats (-10% with respect of SKD), and 5% of carbs (-5% concerning SKD). This diet is useful when you want rapidly lose weight. This type of diet is widely used for practicing bodybuilding because proteins are monomers made of amino acids responsible for building muscle.

CHAPTER 2: BENEFITS OF THE KETO DIET OVER 50s

The ketogenic diet has become very popular because of the success of obtaining results in losing fat and getting healthier. When you start a new diet is always challenging, and you don't know what to expect from it. So now, we are going to have an overview of the pros of this diet. For aging women, menopause will bring severe changes and challenges, but the ketogenic diet can help you switch gears effortlessly to continue enjoying a healthy and happy life. Menopause can upset hormonal levels in women, which consequently affects brainpower and cognitive abilities. Furthermore, due to fewer estrogens and progesterone production, your sex drive declines, and you suffer from sleep issues and mood problems. Let's have a look at how a ketogenic diet will help solve these side effects.

KETO BENEFITS

LOSE WEIGHT

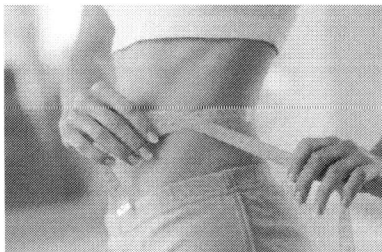

This is maybe the most obvious benefit that the keto diet can do, but if we stop for a moment thinking about the other diets, we can say they are so efficacious as keto is? I will give you the answer: NO. If you think of a regular diet with only a restriction of calories by eating less and with many carbohydrates, when you will stop the diet, it is more likely that you will gain your lose fatback.

With Keto, studies have shown that people have been able to follow this diet and relay fewer hunger pangs and suppressed appetite while losing weight at the same time! With the keto diet, you minimize carbohydrate intake, which brings to more occasional blood sugar spikes. This is very important because the fluctuations in blood sugar levels make you feel hungrier and more prone to snacking in between meals. Instead, by guiding the body towards ketosis, you are eating a more fulfilling diet of fat and protein and harnessing energy from ketone molecules instead of glucose. Studies show that low-carb diets effectively reduce visceral fat (the fat you commonly see around the abdomen increases as you become obese). This reduces your risk of obesity and improves your health in the long run.

REDUCE THE RISK OF HEART-RELATED DISEASE

Now maybe you will think about how the keto diet can help in cardiovascular diseases if it's based on having a high fat intake? Well, research shows that switching to Keto can lower your blood pressure, increase your HDL good cholesterol, and reduce your triglyceride fatty acid levels. That's because the fat you consume with the ketogenic diet is healthy and high-quality fats, so they mitigate many cardiovascular symptoms and the risk of the onset of heart disease. The diet helps boost your HDL cholesterol level in your blood and, at the same time, decrease your LDL cholesterol level ("bad cholesterol"). It also reduces the level of triglyceride fatty acids in the bloodstream, whose top-level in the blood can lead to stroke and heart attack. The ketogenic diet is limiting your carbohydrate intake, favoring the intake of fatty acids. In 2018, researchers found that the Keto diet can improve 22 out of 26 risk factors for cardiovascular heart disease! These factors can be critical to some people, especially those who have a history of heart disease in their family.

REDUCE THE RISK OF TYPE 2 DIABETES

Carbohydrates are polymers made by monomers of sugar; thus, when they are metabolized and absorbed by the intestine, the blood sugar level rise and insulin are produced. This is true for people with no health problems or those who are not predisposed to metabolic disease such as diabetes (genetic susceptibility), who have diabetes or are pre-diabetic. In these cases that I have mentioned, the pancreas is less able or unable at all to produce insulin to lower blood sugar levels.

When you are getting older, the pancreas function can be reduced, thus over 50 years old; you can benefit from the keto diet. In fact, the Keto diet is an excellent option because of the minimal intake of carbohydrates it requires. Instead, you are harnessing most of your calories from fat or protein, which will not cause blood sugar spikes and, ultimately, less pressure on the pancreas to secrete insulin. Many studies have found that diabetes patients who followed the Keto diet lost more weight and eventually reduced their fasting glucose levels. This is good news for patients who wants to stabilize their blood sugar levels and reduce their diabetes medication intake.

BODY'S ENERGY LEVELS RISE UP

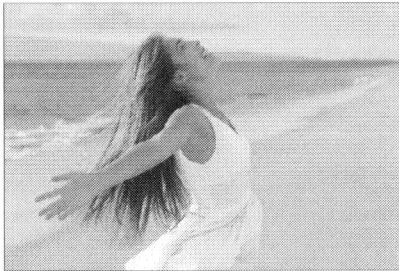

The sources of energy for our body functions are not all the same. Briefly, the carbohydrates are polymers (a chain) made of monomers (a ring of the chain) which are represented by sugar (glucose). When your carbohydrate intake is too high, your "plus" energy is stored by the liver in glycogen form with extra fats, thus getting fat. So, what the Keto diet do to bring more power to your body? The keto diet makes the liver produce ketones using glycogen deposits, thus reducing the stored sugar and fat (glycogen), allowing the weight loss. This makes ketones much more energy-rich and an endless fuel source than glucose, a simple sugar molecule. These ketones can physically and mentally give you a burst of energy, allowing you to have greater focus, clarity, and attention to detail. With nearly 75% of your diet coming from healthy fats, the brain's neural cells and mitochondria have a better energy source to function at the highest level. Some studies have tested patients on the Keto diet and found they had higher cognitive functioning, better memory recall, and less memory loss. The Keto diet can even decrease the occurrence of migraines, which can be very detrimental to patients.

REDUCE RISK OF NEURODEGENERATIVE DISEASES

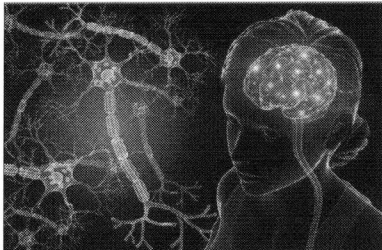

In the 20s, the ketogenic diet was first proposed to combat epilepsy in children. Keto can improve your cognitive functioning level and protect brain cells from injury or damage, thus improving those who suffer from diseases like Alzheimer's or Parkinson's.

How? The ketogenic diet limits carbs intake, reducing blood sugar spikes that the body's neural cells have to keep adjusting to. Studies showed that this neuronal "protection" helps in the prevention of neurodegenerative diseases.

BALANCE YOUR HORMONES

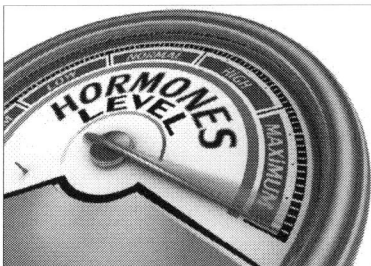

Usually, women face significant symptoms of menopause due to hormonal imbalances. The keto diet for women over 50 works by stabilizing these imbalances such as estrogen, this aids in experiencing fewer and bearable menopausal symptoms like hot flashes. The keto diet also balances blood sugar levels and insulin and helps in controlling insulin sensitivity.

THE SEX DRIVE IS RISING UP

The keto diet surges the absorption of vitamin D, which is essential for enhancing sex drive. Vitamin D ensures stable testosterone levels and other sex hormones that could become unstable due to testosterone levels.

GENERAL INFLAMMATION REDUCTION

Body inflammation is no more than a natural response by the body's immune system; when it becomes uncontrollable, it can lead to an array of health problems, some severe and some minor. The health concerns include acne, autoimmune conditions, arthritis, psoriasis, irritable bowel syndrome, and even acne and eczema. Often, removing sugars and carbohydrates from your diet can help patients with these diseases. Many scientific studies demonstrated that the keto diet decreased a blood marker linked to high inflammation in the body by nearly 40% in the last decades.

INCREASE THE QUALITY OF YOUR SLEEP

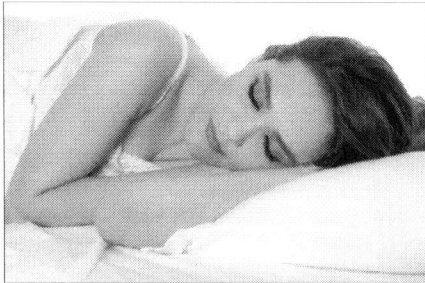

Glucose disturbs your blood sugar levels dramatically, which in turn leads to a low quality of sleep. Along with other menopausal symptoms, good sleep becomes a massive problem as you age. The keto diet for women over 50 not only balances blood glucose levels but also stabilizes other hormones like cortisol, melatonin, and serotonin, warranting an improved and better sleep.

NUTRIENTS REQUIREMENTS

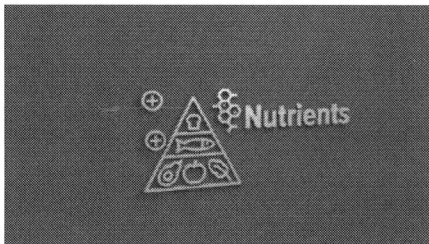

Aging women tend to have higher deficiencies in essential nutrients such as an iron deficiency, which leads to brain fog and fatigue—Vitamin B12 deficiency, which leads to neurological conditions like Dementia. Cognitive impairment in older adults increases the risk of heart disease, cancer development, and cognition, skin, vision, and Vitamin D deficiency due to fats deficiency. On a keto diet, the high-quality proteins ensure adequate and excellent sources of these essential nutrients.

REGULATION OF HORMONES IN WOMEN WHO HAVE PCOS (POLYCYSTIC OVARY SYNDROME) AND PMS (PRE-MENSTRUAL SYNDROME)

Women who have PCOS suffer from infertility problems; hormone regulation is partially driven by insulin blood level; thus, the ketogenic diet can help produce hormones that help in the ovulation process, especially for those women who present PCOS increasing the chance of getting pregnant.

CHAPTER 3: HAVE A DEEPER LOOK TO KETO DIET OVER 50s

WOMEN WHO SUFFER FROM THE FOLLOWING SHOULD NOT ATTEMPT TO EAT LOW CARB WITHOUT THE GUIDANCE OF A HEALTH PROFESSIONAL:

- ✓ Liver of kidney failure
- ✓ Alcohol or drug abuse
- ✓ Type 1 diabetes

- ✓ Pancreatitis
- ✓ Disorders that affect fat metabolism
- ✓ Carnitine deficiency

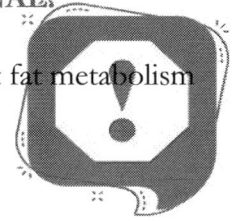

Additionally, women who are pregnant or breastfeeding should avoid eating keto.

THE GENDER AND AGE DIFFERENCE

There are not a lot of keto studies on female subjects. There's still a lot we don't know. Yes, it is possible to reason that lower blood sugar levels and subsequent insulin regulation can prevent diabetes, but it still amounts to guesswork. That being said, the limited studies that have been done found there are significant differences between the two genders and how they react to keto. The main factor that contributes to these dissimilarities comes down to hormones.

HORMONES AND KETO

As a woman, you know that if your hormones are out of balance, your life is too. Hormones are a fundamental part of every process in a woman's body, from reproduction to stress management. It doesn't help that they tend to fluctuate during various times of the month and other reasons, such as a lack of sleep.

Although men have hormones, too, they're not nearly as sensitive to change. And keto is a pretty drastic change, so women have to pay extra attention to how they feel.

WHEN YOU FIRST SWITCH OVER TO EATING LOW CARB, PLEASE TAKE CARE OF:

You may experience a lower sex drive, vaginal dryness, moodiness, and insomnia. This is due to low estrogen levels caused by cutting out processed foods containing soybean oil, which promote estrogen production or menopause. If you want to raise your estrogen levels—which I recommend doing when you're over 50—eat more fat.

Keto may also increase the stress hormone cortisol. When your body realizes it doesn't have enough glucose in its system, it triggers a stress response, and cortisol is released. This chronic stress may lead to an imbalance of blood glucose levels, decreased bone density, and muscle loss. But, considering that eating carbohydrates also causes fluctuating blood sugar levels and a slew of other things, extra cortisol is not the worst that could happen.

THE MENSTRUAL CYCLE

This is another thing women have to face, and men don't. I know you may be thinking about including the menstrual cycle if this book is targeted at women 50 years and older. Well, late-onset menopause is a reality. Some women may continue to menstruate even after the age of 55.

What makes periods extra difficult when you're following keto is the powerful cravings, which makes eating low carb particularly challenging. Other than that, you feel bloated, and you're holding on to more water than usual—this reflects on the scale, which is, in itself, discouraging. You get headaches, which may turn into a keto headache if you don't pay attention to your electrolyte balance and stay hydrated.

Digestion is an issue, and you more than likely feel like eating a bowl of pasta instead of meat and veggies packed with fiber. And then there are the cramps…

This is why so many women fall off the keto bandwagon at that time of the month—something men won't understand.

WHAT YOUR BODY NEEDS AFTER 50

If you're 50, you're most likely in menopause or very close to it; as your hormone levels shift, your body changes. This process is normal and can't be stopped, but if you respond to these changes correctly, it may be slow down!

When you hit the 50-year mark, you may have to aspect some of these changes that we will analyze; then, we will explain how you can use keto to give your body what it needs to stay healthy. Your metabolism will slow down: A slower metabolism means it will take fewer calories for you to gain weight. The high-fat aspect of keto curbs any hunger pangs, and you will automatically eat less to counter a sluggish metabolism.

Hormonal changes may cause digestive issues: Cutting carbohydrates from your diet will promote a healthy gut, which will ease issues like irritable bowel disease or other inflammatory bowel issues.

Bone loss accelerates: The drop in estrogen as you approach or enter menopause is to blame for losing bone density. Exercise will help but eating foods that raise your estrogen levels is also a good idea. The ketogenic diet contains a lot of these foods, among them kale and olives. Your body stores fatter: Fat, protein, and enough fiber will kill any cravings you have and make it easier to avoid temptation. If you don't eat in excess, there won't be fat for your body to hold on to. Your skin changes: Bone broth is an excellent collagen source, which helps your skin maintain its elasticity. Your libido declines: Removing sugary foods and carbs from your diet will help boost your sex drive.

Calcium deficiency becomes a reality: The ketogenic diet allows you to eat dairy, but furthermore, kale, and broccoli, which are stapled low-carb veggies, are high in calcium. A lot of what we experience as we grow older isn't pleasant, but it is in our power to not only make it more bearable but to slow the whole process down.

It's already evident that following a wholesome, nutritious diet will prolong your life by eliminating and preventing dangerous diseases. But calorie restriction also has the ability not only to increase your life but your lifespan. Here's how.

In 2018 a research study was conducted by Redman et al.[1]: participants were asked to eat 15% fewer calories for two years. After the time elapsed, researchers found that not only were their metabolisms slower (meaning their bodies were more energy efficient), but they also had less oxidative stress. Cutting calories can even reduce your risk of getting age-related diseases. It all comes down to slowing your basal metabolism. According to Redman and associates, if a person's metabolism is slow, energy is spent more economically, which means cells and organs can 'work' less, increasing their longevity. Although other factors, such as oxidative stress and dietary and biological elements that influence your metabolism, cutting calories is an excellent way to get it where healthy aging is possible.

KETOGENIC CHALLENGES AFTER 50

It's no wonder that your body will react adversely when you first start keto; cutting carbs from your diet turns everything upside down. All of a sudden has to learn to use ketones as fuel instead of glucose. So, during this transition, you may not feel your greatest. Almost everyone who starts keto experiences some or all of these symptoms:

✓ Nausea	✓ Irritability	✓ Dizziness
✓ Fatigue	✓ Lack of motivation	✓ Keto rash
✓ Headache	✓ Sugar cravings	✓ Constipation
✓ Keto flu	✓ Brain fog	✓ Diarrhea

But, since you're a woman over 50, you may have to face some extra stumbling blocks, chiefly: Your weight loss plateaus: If this happens, up to your fat consumption to the 80% mark. Hormone imbalances: Don't restrict your calories too much, and don't lose too much weight. A woman's body is healthiest, with 22 to 29 percent body fat. Another way to combat these pesky hormones is to sync your diet with your menstrual cycle. When your period starts, eat more protein, then from days 6 to 11, go to the end of low carb, and on days 12 to 16, eat a lot of avocados, broccoli, garlic, and parsley. You can end your cycle (days 17 to 28) by eating moderate low carb.

[1]Redman LM et al., 2018. *Cell Metab.* doi:10.1016/j.cmet.2018.02.019

CHAPTER 4. DIET & EXERCISE: AN IMPORTANT LIFESTYLE

BENEFITS EXERCISING FOR OVER 50

You may say "Am I too old for exercise?!," there is nothing more wrong with that! I will explain to you why:

REGULAR EXERCISE PREVENTS DISEASES

Generally speaking, regular physical activity has been known to reduce the risks of diseases such as diabetes and heart disease.

This is truer for seniors who are often immunocompromised, and exercising can improve your body's overall immune functioning and strength against bone fracture and other kinds of age-related issues. Even if you can't hit the gym, some light exercise can play an integral role in disease management.

SOCIALIZATION AND COMMUNITY

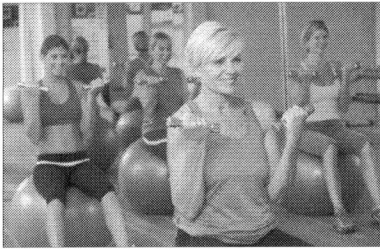

Aging can be a daunting process, but it becomes fun when a community surrounds you. Opting for yoga or fitness classes not only makes exercising more fun but also helps you strengthen social ties with other older adults in your neighborhood. It can help ward off the occasional loneliness that one is likely to feel at old age. Plus, this will help you stay committed to your goals and lead a healthier lifestyle. Regular exercise also improves your cognitive function, reducing the risk of dementia.

EXERCISES FOR OVER 50: TIPS & TRICKS

Here I want to give some ideas and tips for exercises you can enjoy:

LIGHT WEIGHT TRAINING

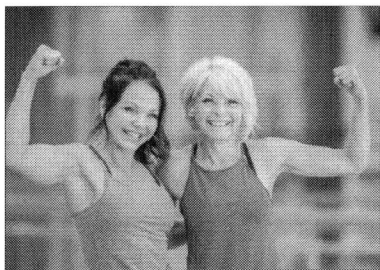

You can start with some weight training to build muscle mass and maintain bone density. If you're more interested in working out at home rather than going to the gym, perform arm lifts and shoulder presses.

Ideally, you'll want to join a fitness center or gym where you can meet like-minded people. You can also get a personal trainer who can guide workouts tailored to you. Either way, remember to take it easy at first because you don't want to push yourself too hard. Again, you won't have to lift 150 pounds on the bench. Weight training is still a crucial exercise at any age because you'll always have to lift, move, and put things down. You just need to reduce the number of weights you lift to compensate for your lack of muscle mass and strength.

There is no definitive starting point here. You need to explore where your limit lies, so start light and work your way up to heavier weights. Aim for a weight that is just light enough to allow you to do 10 reps where the last few reps become challenging. Increase the weight when you can do more than 10 reps. If you can't reach 10 reps, drop the weight.

Lifting weights will help you build muscle to compensate for lost mass and keep your body healthy. Try to work out twice a week for each muscle group to keep the muscle evenly strengthened throughout your body.

Other than that, there are a few things you need to pay attention to. Don't exercise the same muscle group two days in a row. Give it time to rest because it only gets stronger when you rest after an exercise. Also, if you feel pain, stop or try a lighter weight.

Alternatively, if barbells and dumbbells seem intimidating to you, you can try the following:

- ✓ Resistance bands
- ✓ Exercise equipment
- ✓ Push-ups
- ✓ Modified squats and lunges

SQUATS & SIT-UPS

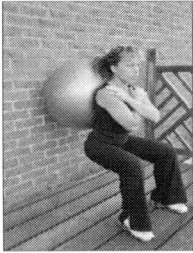

When you're working on a workout program, you shouldn't skip the idea of strength training. Squats are an excellent way to strengthen your lower body muscles. Doing squats is relatively easy, and you won't need any kind of equipment, except maybe a chair to support you. You can also use an exercise ball behind your back to increase the level of difficulty. However, if you have balance or knee problems, we recommend skipping this exercise and opting for something much easier.

YOGA

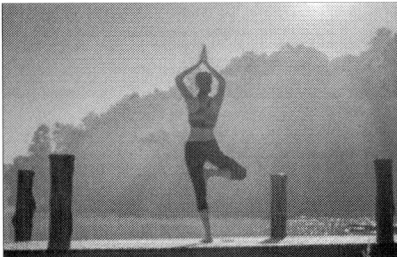

Yoga is relaxing, healthy, and can be enjoyed with a group. It helps improve the flexibility of your joints. Some classic yoga poses you may want to try to include the seated forward bend, downward-facing dog, and warrior. It also allows seniors to stay flexible and maintain their sense of balance. If you have trouble moving or stretching, you can try chair yoga.

SWIMMING

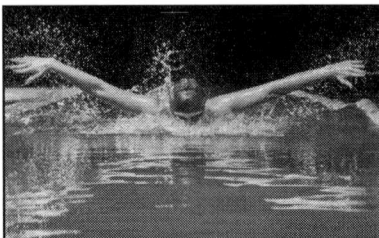

Do you find regular exercise too dull? Swimming is a fun, non-impact exercise that can get you through the day. The water offers gentle resistance while also giving you a cardiovascular workout. It also builds muscle capacity and helps you build strength again. It's almost painless and doesn't bother your aging joints. Swimming offers an endurance workout and will also help you get back on your feet.

AEROBICS

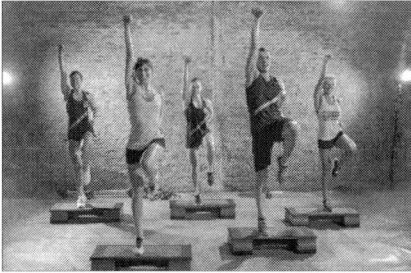

Participating in an aerobics class can significantly help you maintain your healthy muscles and mobility. It will improve your balance and reduce your risk of falls, thus dramatically improving your life's overall quality as you age. Many studies have also indicated how aerobic exercises can protect memory, sharpen the mind, and improve older adults' cognitive function. If you don't feel comfortable participating in a class, you'll find many videos online. Aerobic exercises are also known to get the heart pumping, improving cardiovascular aid.

WALKING

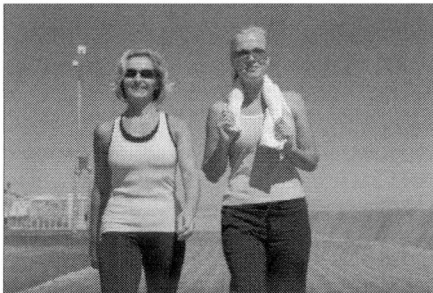

If bodybuilding isn't your thing, old-fashioned walking should do the trick too. Consider taking a nice walk around your neighborhood or going to a nearby park. You'll be able to enjoy the weather and, why not, meet some friends while you do it.

If you prefer to work out at home, wear a pedometer, walk around the house, or use the stairs or a step stool. Move your arms and lift your knees as you take each step to increase your workout.

CYCLING

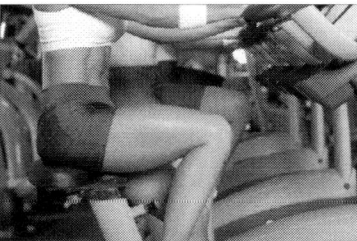

Cycling is just as easy on your joints. It helps lower your risk of heart attacks, regulate your blood pressure, and help your mood. Pedaling is quite useful if you have back, neck, or shoulder pain if you use a stationary recumbent bike. Such a device is very ergonomically comfortable because you can rest your arms and back in a comfortable position while moving your legs.

Of course, to get the full benefit of cycling, you should visit the bike paths. As an added benefit, you can enjoy the beautiful natural landscape.

PILATES

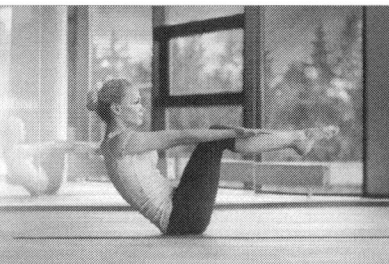

Perform exercises that strengthen the core of your back, especially if you feel pain in your back. In this case, Pilates will work wonders on your body. Simply put, Pilates is all about building long, lean muscles and conditioning your body using controlled movements. It strengthens, stretches, and tones all core and stabilization areas while increasing flexibility, range of motion, and perfecting posture. Besides, Pilates is very easy to practice because there are alternative exercises to help beginners, especially stiff limbs.

CHAPTER 5. TIPS ON LOSING WEIGHT OVER 50s

PROCRASTINATION COULD BE YOUR FRIEND!

Eating chips, crackers, or any other salty snack can make you eat too quickly. The problem is that giving up these delicious cold turkey-style snacks is difficult, especially if you've developed a taste for them. What do you do? Well, remove these foods from your home immediately. Limit food in the house for the week or only have healthy snacks in the house. Even when you have a sudden craving for unhealthy snacks, the inconvenience of going out to buy one is enough to deter you and help you suppress hunger. Another solution is to tell yourself that you will get that unhealthy snack "tomorrow." We are procrastinators for nature, so use that to your advantage as well. When you set up a "plan" like that, your mind is tricked into thinking that you'll do it when the time is right, even if that time never comes. But what if you need to go out shopping for next week's keto meals? You have two options. You can go to the grocery store carrying only enough money to get everything you need for next week's meals. This way, you simply can't afford to buy extra snacks. But this requires your prior knowledge of the prices of the products you need to buy, and any price change can leave you with a few extra pennies or not enough money. To get around this problem, I recommend only bringing a little extra cash if there are price changes. An alternative I like is to bring someone with you for the trip, but let them carry all the money. The amount is not significant here, but it does require the other person to be firm in not letting you buy that fry. They have the money, and they will have to stick to the plan of buying enough for the week, nothing more. It will be a little uncomfortable for the other person, but it should help you stay on top of things.

EAT LESS AT NIGHT

Breakfast is the most important meal of the day, considering you haven't eaten in the last 8 hours, while the interval between breakfast and lunch and between lunch and dinner is 5 or 6 hours at most. Dinner should be small because your body doesn't need to expend that much energy when you're sleeping anyway. So the excess energy becomes fat. So, keep your dinner light. For one thing, it helps you lose weight. Another reason is that if you have a heavy dinner, your body will struggle to digest everything. This means that your body will stay active until all the food has been digested, which means you won't get a night of restful sleep if you can sleep at all. Bottom line: Eat light and eat dinner at least 4 hours before you go to bed. Any earlier, and you'll have a hard time sleeping.

GET ENOUGH SLEEP

When you're over 50, you no longer have the ability to party past midnight without feeling extremely tired for the rest of the month. If there's a crucial time to get 8 hours of sleep a day, it's right now. Getting enough sleep helps your body regulate the hormones in your body, so try to aim for 7-9 hours of sleep a day. You can get more restful sleep by creating a nightly routine of not looking at your computer, phone, or TV screen for at least 1 hour before bed. You can drink warm milk or water to help your body relax, or even do 10 to 20 min. of stretching to get a restful sleep. While we're on the topic of sleep, try to keep a consistent sleep schedule. I understand that you want to sleep in and wake up 1 to 4 hours later than usual on the weekends. But if you want to go to bed and wake up at the same time, your mood and energy level will be higher. Another benefit is that your body will learn to wake up on its own, even without an alarm clock.

FIND AN ACTIVITY YOU ENJOY

When you get enough exercise, you will know what activities you enjoy. One way to encourage yourself to exercise more regularly is to make it fun rather than a chore. If possible, stick to your favorite activities, and you can get the most out of your exercises. Keep in mind that the activities you enjoy may not be useful or necessary, so you need to find other practices to compensate for not enjoying them as much. For example, if you like jogging, you can work your leg muscles, but your arms are not involved. So, you need to do push-ups or other strength training exercises. Here, your trainer can help you decide and create a workout routine that you can stick to.

MINDFUL EATING

Mindfulness is not limited to meditation alone. Again, we won't go over meditation in this book because that's another topic altogether. But what you can do here is learn to love and appreciate your food. It sounds obnoxious, but it helps your mood and promotes weight loss. In a nutshell, you just need to put your phone away and remove any other source of distraction and focus solely on your food, how it tastes, etc. This means eating slowly. You will learn to appreciate how tasty your food is because you are focusing on eating. How does this translate to weight loss? You see, there is a system in your body that determines how full you are. The problem is that this system is not instantaneous. It takes a while to measure how full your stomach is before sending the signal to your brain. So, when you eat too fast, you have already gone a mile by the time you feel full. If you eat slowly, your body has enough time to register your fullness bite by bite. Thus, when you feel full, you have not overeaten.

CONVENIENCE FOODS? ANSWER NO!

Convenience foods are convenient but not healthy. Not by a long shot. They're high in calories and often don't contain essential nutrients like protein, fiber, vitamins, etc. If you can, avoid convenience foods altogether.

COOK AT HOME MORE

Or eat out less frequently. Why should you do this? First, surely you know that only a few places serve keto foods, let alone those that follow your diet plan. You have to prepare your food if you want to go on a keto diet. Another advantage is the economy. You will buy most of your ingredients and prepare your meals ahead of time. This means you'll only spend your money on the ingredients you know you'll need.

Consider incorporating more produce into your diet, some of which I have already covered. Consider that eating fruits and vegetables is full of nutrients your body needs to stay healthy; remember to include them in your diet.

I WILL NEVER STOP TO SAY: HYDRATE PROPERLY!

This means drinking enough water or herbal tea and not drinking sugary drinks or other beverages that contain sugar. Making the transition will be difficult for the first few weeks, but your body will thank you for it. There's nothing healthier than good old plain water, and the recommended amount is 2 liters a day. However, since you're on a keto diet, your body needs to consume more water, so consider 2 gallons the absolute minimum amount of water you need to drink. I recommend drinking between 3 or even 4 gallons a day when you're on a keto diet. If you're thirsty, then that's a sign of dehydration, so drink some water. Drinking lots of water also leads to more calories burned. You can shave off a few more calories by drinking cold water because your body will spend more energy trying to regulate your body temperature.

CHECK WITH A HEALTHCARE PROVIDER AND TALK TO A DIETITIAN

The first thing you should do before getting into any diet is to consult your dietitian. While the keto diet works for many people, you never really know if it will work for you. Therefore, it is wise to ask your dietitian first before you jump in, rather than suffer some adverse effects because your body is not compatible with this diet.

The keto diet works for many people, but it isn't for everyone. Your dietitian can tell you whether the keto diet would work. Before starting the diet, check in with your healthcare provider to ensure that you do not have any medical condition that prevents you from losing weight, such as hypothyroidism and polycystic ovarian syndrome. It helps to know well in advance whether your body is even capable of losing fat in the first place before you commit and see no result, right?

MOVE MORE AND HIRE A PERSONAL TRAINER

While we're still talking about exercise, consider getting a personal trainer. Your trainer will also be an exercise partner because they will keep you accountable to your schedule. Your trainer is helpful when you're doing strength training because they can teach you how to perform the exercise, preventing you from hurting yourself properly.

Moving doesn't necessarily mean more cardio exercises. You can't expect to achieve more effective weight loss if you exercise for 30 min. a day and then sit in a chair for the rest of the day. The idea is to burn more calories than you can take in, so it pays to be a little more active throughout the day. If you have an office job, consider getting up at least once an hour and taking a short break by walking around the lobby for at least 5 min. It doesn't sound like much, but it helps in the long run.

YOUR BODY ISN'T JUST "WEIGHT" ALONE!

Your body is made up of fat, muscle, fluid, bone, etc. What you want to lose is fat weight, not muscle or fluid weight. You want as little fat mass in your body as possible while maintaining a healthy level of non-fat mass in your body. There are many ways to measure your body fat, but the easiest method is to measure your calves, thighs, waist, chest, and biceps.

PROTEIN ASSUMPTION

Protein is essential for weight loss and youthfulness, including protection against muscle breakdown and other aging disorders. Combine a high protein intake with strength training, and you can be sure you'll build muscle faster than it can degrade. You won't look like Arnold when he was a bodybuilder, but you may well look fitter than the 20-year-old guy in your workplace.

SUPPLEMENTS: WHAT I NEED

As you age, your body begins to lose the ability to absorb certain nutrients, which leads to deficits. For example, vitamin B12 and folate are among the most common nutrients lacking in people over 50. They have an impact on mood, energy level, and rate of weight loss. Therefore, if you feel tired when following the keto diet, you may not be getting enough of the nutrients your body needs. This doesn't mean you should eat more, no. You just need to take the right supplements.

VERY IMPORTANT

Remember that staying hydrated, especially when you are first starting your ketogenic diet! Your safest bet is to always **stick with water**. Whether you like your water sparkling or flat, this is still going to be a zero-carb option. If you are struggling with a headache or the keto fly, remember that you can always throw a dash of salt in there.

Here is a tip:

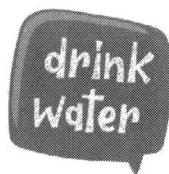

UNSWEETENED COFFEE AND TEA

These two drinks are carb-free, so long as you don't add sugar, milk, or other sweeteners. Both contain caffeine that improves your metabolism and suppresses your appetite. A word of warning to those who love light coffee and tea lattes, though. They are made with non-fat milk and contain a lot of carbs.

CHAPTER 6: KETO FRIENDLY FOODS

It's time to learn what you can and cannot eat while following the ketogenic diet. Up to this point, you have most likely followed the food pyramid that states the importance of fruits and vegetables. While they will still be necessary for vitamins and nutrients, you will need to be selective.

You'll find a complete list of foods you can enjoy on the keto diet here!

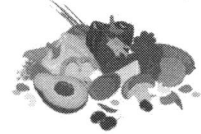

VEGETABLES & FRUITS

Vegetables can be tricky when starting the ketogenic diet. Some vegetables contain more carbohydrates than others. Remember: Vegetables that grow above the ground are good; below ground is terrible.

Some popular above-ground vegetables that you should consider for your diet (starting with the least carbs to the most carbs) include:

✓ Spinach	✓ Tomato	✓ Green Beans
✓ Lettuce	✓ Eggplant	✓ Broccoli
✓ Avocado	✓ Cabbage	✓ Peppers
✓ Asparagus	✓ Zucchini	✓ Brussel Sprouts
✓ Olives	✓ Cauliflower	
✓ Cucumber	✓ Kale	

Vegetables you should avoid:

✓ Carrots	✓ Beetroot	✓ Sweet Potato
✓ Onion	✓ Rutabaga	
✓ Parsnip	✓ Potato	

Every food you put on your plate includes three macronutrients: fat, protein, and carbohydrates. This will be an essential lesson to learn before you start your keto diet, so be sure to take your time to learn how to calculate them.

The golden rule is that meat and dairy are primarily composed of protein and fat. Vegetables are mostly carbohydrates. Remember that less than 5% of your calories should come from carbohydrates while following the ketogenic diet. This is probably the most challenging task to accomplish when you first start; there are hidden carbs everywhere! You'll be amazed at how quickly 20g of carbs will be gone in a single day, much less in a single meal! When you first start, you may want to dip your toes into the carb cut. As a rule, vegetables that have less than five net carbs can be eaten reasonably freely. To make them a little more ketogenic, I suggest putting butter on the veggies to have a fat source in the meal.

If you still struggle at the store, figuring out which vegetables are ketogenic, look for vegetables with leaves. Vegetables that have left are typically spinach and lettuce, both of which are keto-friendly. Another rule to follow is to look for green vegetables. Generally, green vegetables like green peppers and green cabbage are lower in carbs!

Much like vegetables, some berries and fruits contain hidden carbohydrates. As a general rule, the more considerable the amount of fruit, the more sugar it has; this is why fruit is seen as nature's candy! On the ketogenic diet, this is a no-go. While berries are fine in moderation, it's best to leave other fruits out for the best results.

You may be asking yourself, do I need to eat fruit for the nutrients? The truth is, you can get the same nutrients from vegetables while costing fewer carbs on the ketogenic diet. While eating a few berries now and then won't get you out of ketosis, it's good to see how they affect you. But, if you feel like indulging in fruit as a treat, you can try some of the following: Raspberries, blackberries, strawberries, plums, kiwis, cherries, blueberries, clementines, cantaloupe, peaches.

Most vegetables contain many nutrients that your body can benefit from significantly, even though they are low in calories and carbohydrates. Also, some of them contain fiber, which helps with bowel movement. Also, your body spends more energy breaking down and digesting fiber-rich food, so it helps with weight loss.

Let's look at some of them more specifically:

AVOCADOS

Avocados are so popular nowadays in the health community that people associate the word "health" with avocados. They are full of vitamins and minerals such as potassium. Also, avocados have been proven to help the body go into ketosis faster.

BERRIES

Many fruits contain too many carbohydrates making them unsuitable in a keto diet, but not berries. They are low in carbs and high in fiber. Some of the best berries to include in your diet are blackberries, blueberries, raspberries, and strawberries.

SHIRATAKI NOODLES

If you love noodles and pasta but don't want to give them up, then shirataki noodles are the perfect alternative. They are rich in water and contain much fiber, which means low carbs and calories and hunger suppression.

OILS AND OTHER FATS

The key to getting enough fat in your diet will depend on the sauces and oils you use for cooking on the ketogenic diet. When you put enough fat in your meals, it will keep you satisfied after each meal. The key here is to pay attention to the labels. You may be surprised to learn that some of your favorite condiments may have hidden sugars (looking at you, ketchup).

While you may have to be a little more careful with your condiments, you can never go wrong with butter! Up until this point, you've probably been encouraged to eat a low-fat diet. Now, I want you to embrace the fat! You can put butter in just about anything! Put butter on your veggies, put it in your coffee, and be creative!

Oils, on the other hand, can be a little more complicated. You can use natural oils like fish oil, sesame oil, almond oil, ghee, pure olive oil, and even peanut oil. What you want to avoid are oils that have been created in the last sixty years or so. You want to avoid oils, including soybean oil, corn oil, sunflower oil, and any vegetable oil. Unfortunately, these oils have been highly processed and can hinder your process.

Stick with these for your diet instead:

- ✓ Butter
- ✓ Vinaigrette
- ✓ Coconut Oil
- ✓ Mayo
- ✓ Mustard
- ✓ Guacamole
- ✓ Heavy Cream
- ✓ Thousand Island Dressing
- ✓ Salsa
- ✓ Blue Cheese Dressing
- ✓ Ranch Dip
- ✓ Pesto

When it comes to dairy, high-fat will be your best option. Cheese and butter are great options, but keep yogurts in moderation. When it comes to milk, you'll want to avoid it because there is extra sugar in the milk. If you like heavy cream, this can be excellent for your cooking but should be used sparingly in your coffee.

Let's look at some of them more specifically:

COCONUT OIL

Coconut oil and other coconut-related products such as coconut milk and coconut powder are perfect for a keto diet. Coconut oil contains mainly MCTs that are converted to ketones by the liver for use as an immediate source of energy.

OLIVE OIL

Olive oil is very beneficial to your heart because it contains oleic acid, which helps decrease heart disease risk factors. Extra virgin olive oil (EVO) is also rich in antioxidants. Best of all, olive oil can be used as a primary source, and it has no carbohydrates. The same goes for olive.

BUTTER AND CREAM

These two foods contain many fats and a minimal amount of carbohydrates, making them an excellent option for your keto diet.

NUTS AND SEEDS

When you start the ketogenic diet, you will be able to eat as many nuts as you want because they are high in fat. While you can enjoy a healthy portion of nuts, you can overdo it with nuts. As with fruits and vegetables, you would be surprised to know that there are hidden carbohydrates here too!

Nuts and seeds are also low in carbs but high in fat. They are also healthy and have lots of nutrients and fiber. They help reduce heart disease, cancer, depression, and other disease risks. The fiber in these also helps make you feel full longer, so you'd consume fewer calories, and your body would spend more calories digesting them.

The nuts with the lowest carbohydrate content are macadamia nuts, Brazil nuts, and pecans. These are relatively low in carbohydrates and can be enjoyed freely while following the ketogenic diet. If you are looking for a healthy, these are all great ketogenic snack options or something to throw in your salad.

When you're at the store, you'll want to avoid nuts that have been treated with frostings and sugars. All of these extras add sugar and carbs, which you'll want to avoid. Nuts with more carbohydrates include cashews, pistachios, almonds, pine nuts, and peanuts. It would be best to avoid these nuts.

The problem with eating nuts is that it's easy to overdo it with them. While they are technically keto-friendly, they still contain a high number of calories. With that in mind, you should only eat them when you are hungry and in need of energy. On the ketogenic diet, you'll want to avoid snacking between meals. You don't need nuts, but they taste good! If you plan on losing weight, put down the nuts and choose a healthier snack instead.

MEAT, FISH, EGG AND CHEESE

On the ketogenic diet, the meat will become a staple for you! When choosing your meats, try to stick to organic, grass-fed, and unprocessed. I want you to keep in mind that the ketogenic diet is not meant to be high in protein; it is high in fat. People often link the ketogenic diet to a high-meat diet, and that's not true. At the beginning of the diet, you don't need to have excessive amounts of meat or protein. If you have extra protein, it will be converted to glucose, throwing you out of ketosis.

Meat and poultry are the staple foods of most keto diets. Most keto meals revolve around these two ingredients. This is because they contain no carbohydrates and contain many vitamins and minerals. Besides, they are a great source of protein.

There are several proteins that you can enjoy while following the ketogenic diet. When it comes to beef, you will want to do your best to stick to the fattier cuts. Some of the best cuts include ground beef, roast beef, veal, and steak. If poultry is more your style, look for the darker, fattier meats. Some good poultry selection options would be game, turkey, duck, quail, and good old chicken. Other options include:

- ✓ Pork loin
- ✓ Tenderloin
- ✓ Pork chops
- ✓ Ham
- ✓ Bacon

With your ketogenic diet, you'll also enjoy a variety of seafood dishes! At the store, you'll want to look for wild-caught sources. Some of the best options include mahi-mahi, catfish, cod, halibut, trout, sardines, salmon, tuna, and mackerel. If shellfish is more your style, you can enjoy lobster, muscles, crab, clams, and even oysters!

Keep in mind that when selecting your meat, try to avoid cured meats and processed meats. These items, such as jerky, hot dogs, salami, and pepperoni, have many artificial ingredients, additives, and unnecessary sugars that will prevent you from achieving ketosis. Now you know the best options. Stick with them!

EGGS

Eggs make up most of the foods you will eat on a keto diet because they are the healthiest and most versatile food of all. Even a large egg contains very few carbohydrates but contains much protein, making it a perfect keto diet option. Besides, eggs have been shown to have an appetite-suppressing effect, making you feel full longer and regulating blood sugar levels. This leads to a lower calorie intake for about a day. Just be sure to eat the whole egg because the nutrients are in the yolk.

SEAFOOD

Fish and shellfish are perfect for keto diets. Many fish are rich in B vitamins, potassium, and selenium. Salmon, sardines, mackerel, and other fatty fish also contain lots of omega-3 fats that help regulate insulin levels. These are so low in carbohydrates that it is negligible.

Shellfish are a different story because some contain few carbohydrates, while others have many. Shrimp and most crabs are fine, but watch out for other types of crustaceans.

PLAIN GREEK YOGURT AND COTTAGE CHEESE

These two foods are high in protein and a small number of carbs, small enough to include in your keto diet. They also help suppress your appetite by making you feel full for a long time, and they can be eaten alone and still be delicious.

CHEESE

Milk, as I will discuss in the next chapter, is not acceptable. You can get away with cheese, though. Cheese is delicious and nutritious. Luckily, although hundreds of cheese types are all low in carbs and full of fat, eating cheese can even help your muscles and slow down aging.

...AND SNACKs?

The answer is yes, but in moderation. If you're looking for something to grab, look for easy whole foods; some of these basics include eggs, cheese, deli meats, avocados, and even olives. As long as you have these staple foods in your fridge, this should keep you from reaching for the high-carb foods.

Vegetable sticks are crunchy and always a great option! There are plenty of dipping sauces to add fat to your meal. Also, pork rinds are a delicious zero-carb treat. Dried meat is also a good option, as long as you know how many carbs are in a commercial package.

With the right options in mind, it's always good to take a look at the bad ones. When snacking, avoid high-carb fruits, coffee with cream and sugar juices. Before you started the ketogenic diet, these were probably the most comfortable option. You'll also want to avoid the obvious candy, chips, and donuts. Just remember that when you're selecting your foods, ask yourself whether or not it's fueling you.

Let's look at some of them more specifically:

DARK CHOCOLATE AND COCOA POWDER

These two foods are delicious and contain antioxidants. Dark chocolate is associated with reducing the risk of heart disease by lowering blood pressure. Just be sure to choose only dark chocolate with at least 70% cocoa solids.

CHAPTER 7: KETO UNFRIENDLY FOODS

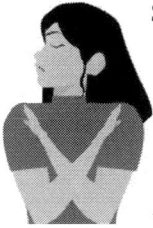

Some of the food you avoid is even healthy, but they just contain too many carbs. Here is a list of typical food you should limit or avoid altogether:

CEREAL

Cereal is also a big culprit because sugary breakfast cereals contain a lot of carbohydrates. This goes for "healthy cereals" as well. Just because they use other words to describe their product doesn't mean you should believe them. This also applies to oatmeal, whole grain cereals, etc.

By the time you eat a bowl of cereal when you're on the keto diet, you're already well over your carb limit, and we haven't even added milk into the equation! Therefore, avoid whole grains or the cereals we mention here altogether.

GLUTEN-FREE BAKED GOODS

Wheat, barley, and rye all contain gluten. Some people who have celiac disease still want to enjoy these goodies, but they can't because their intestines become inflamed in response to gluten. For this reason, gluten-free variations have been created to meet their needs. Gluten-free diets are all the rage these days, but many people don't seem to realize that they contain quite a few carbs. This includes gluten-free bread, muffins, and other baked goods. They contain even more carbs than their gluten-free variant. Also, the flour used to make these gluten-free products is made from grains and starches. When you consume gluten-free bread, your blood sugar levels spike.

So, limit yourself to whole grain foods. Alternatively, you can use almond or coconut flour to make your low carb bread.

BREAD, GRAINS & PASTA

Bread is a staple food in many countries. There are loaves of bread, bagels, tortillas, and the list goes on. However, no matter what form bread takes, it is still full of carbohydrates. The same goes for whole grains as well because they are made from refined flour. Depending on your daily carb limit, eating a sandwich or bagel can put you over your daily limit. So, if you want to eat bread, it's best to make keto variations at home instead. Grains like rice, wheat, and oats also contain a lot of carbs. Limit or avoid that as well.

Pasta is also a staple food in many countries. It is versatile and convenient. Like any other convenient food, pasta is high in carbohydrates. When you are on your keto diet, spaghetti or any other type of pasta is not recommended. You can probably get away with eating a small portion, but that's not an option.

Luckily, this doesn't mean you have to give it up altogether. If you're craving pasta, you can try other low-carb options like spiralized vegetables or shirataki noodles

BEANS AND LEGUMES

They are also very nutritious because they are high in fiber. Research has shown that eating them has many health benefits, such as reducing inflammation and heart disease risk. However, they are also high in carbohydrates. You may be able to enjoy a small amount of them when you are on your keto diet, but make sure you know exactly how much you can eat before you exceed your carb limit.

VEGETABLES & FRUITS

Vegetables are just as healthy for your body. Most keto diets do not care how many vegetables you eat, as long as they are low in starch. Vegetables that are high in fiber can help with weight loss. For one, they make you feel full longer, so they help suppress your appetite. Another benefit is that your body burns more calories to break down and digest. They also help control blood sugar and aid bowel movements.

Fruits are healthy for you. They have been linked to a lower risk of heart disease and cancer. However, there are some that you need to avoid in your keto diets. The problem is that some of these foods contain a lot of carbohydrates, such as bananas, raisins, dates, mangoes, and pears. As a general rule, avoid sweet and dried fruits. Berries are an exception because they don't contain as much sugar and are high in fiber. You can still eat some, about 50 grams. Moderation is key. But that also means you should avoid or limit high-starch vegetables because they have more carbohydrates than fiber. This includes corn, potatoes, sweet potatoes, and beets.

LOW-FAT AND FAT-FREE SALAD DRESSINGS

As mentioned earlier, fruits and vegetables are mostly fine, as long as they're low in carbs. But if you have to buy salads, keep in mind that commercial dressings contain more carbs than you think, especially the fat-free and low-fat variants. So, if you want to enjoy your salad, dress it with a creamy, high-fat dressing instead. To cut down on the carbs, you can use vinegar and olive oil, both of which have been shown to be beneficial for heart health and weight loss.

JUICE & BEER

Juices are perhaps the worst drink you can put in your system when you are on a keto diet. You can argue that the juice provides some nutrients, but the problem is that it contains many carbohydrates that are very easy to digest. As a result, your blood sugar level will spike every time you drink it. This is also true for vegetable juices because of the fast-digesting carbohydrates present. Another problem is that the brain does not process liquid carbohydrates in the same way as solid carbohydrates. Solid carbs can help suppress your appetite, but liquid carbs will only put your appetite into overdrive.

In fact, you can drink most alcoholic beverages in moderation without fear. For example, dry wine doesn't have many carbs, and hard liquor doesn't have any at all. So you can drink them without worry. Beer is an exception to this rule because it contains a lot of carbohydrates. Carbohydrates in beer or other liquids are considered liquid carbohydrates, and they are even more dangerous than solid carbohydrates. You see, when you eat carbohydrate-rich food, you at least feel full. When you drink liquid carbohydrates, you don't feel full as quickly, so there is a little appetite-suppressing effect.

SWEETENED YOGURT & MILK

Yogurt is very healthy because it is tasty and doesn't have a lot of carbohydrates. It is a very versatile food to have in your keto diet. The problem comes when you consume carbohydrate-rich yogurt variations, such as fruit, low-fat, sweetened, or fat-free yogurt. A single serving of sweetened yogurt contains as many carbs as a single serving of dessert.

If you love yogurt, you can get away with half a cup of plain Greek yogurt with 50 grams of raspberries or blackberries. I mentioned earlier that cereal contains many carbs, and a breakfast cereal will put you way over your carb limit without you adding milk. Milk also has a lot of carbs on its own. Therefore, avoid it if you can, even though milk is a good source of many nutrients like calcium, potassium, and other B vitamins.

Of course, this doesn't mean you have to give up milk completely. You can get away with a tbsp. or two of milk for your coffee. But cream or half-and-half is better if you drink coffee frequently. These two contain very few carbohydrates. But if you love to drink milk in large quantities or need it to make your favorite drinks, consider using unsweetened coconut or almond milk instead.

SUGAR

We mean sugar in any form, including honey. You may already be aware of what foods that contain a lot of sugar, such as cookies, candy, and cakes, are banned on a keto diet or any other form of diet that is designed to lose weight.

You may not know that natural sugar, such as honey, is just as high in carbohydrates as processed sugar. Raw forms of sugar contain even more carbohydrates.

Not only is sugar, in general, high in carbs, but it also adds little to no nutritional value to your meal. When you're on a keto diet, you need to keep in mind that your diet will consist of high fiber and nutrients. Sugar is out of the question!

If you want to sweeten your food, you can use a healthy sweetener instead of adding as many carbohydrates to your food.

CHAPTER 4: FAQ: KETO CHALLENGES AFTER 50

→ DOES KETO DIET HAVE SIDE EFFECTS?

It would be irresponsible to ignore the side effects. Some possible adverse effects could occur once you start the ketogenic diet. All types of diets have adverse effects, to begin with because your body has become accustomed to bad habits. Once you switch to a more positive way of eating, your body goes into a sort of rebellion phase, so it feels like everything is going wrong. For example, a person who used to eat a lot of sugar in a day may have severe headaches once they start avoiding sugar. This is a symptom of withdrawal and tells you that your diet is making positive changes in the body - the important thing is to know why my body is reacting this way!

→ WHY SOME PEOPLE HAVE FLU WHEN STARTED KETOGENIC DIET?

Symptoms include pain, fatigue, cramping, rashes, and diarrhea. It can be experienced, especially during the first few days on a keto diet. This can be caused by dehydration due to your body losing a lot of water and electrolytes. When your energy comes from fat instead of protein, your body tends to lose more electrolytes and water through urination. This loss is further accelerated by the low insulin and muscle glycogen levels that accompany the keto diet. Most ketogenic diets consist of food with low water and potassium levels, accelerating the body's loss of water and electrolytes.

What can I do? You can manage the keto flu by drinking lots of water. You can also eat lots of soup. If you get enough rest, you will give your body enough energy to fight the flu independently.

It would be helpful to lower the effects of the flu by getting enough sleep. You can also drink plenty of water to minimize the impact of keto flu. Some supplements can be found in natural sources such as organic coffee or matcha tea to help you overcome the flu. Make sure you have enough salts and electrolytes as well.

→ WHY I HAVE DIFFICULTIES IN BREATH? AND HOW CAN BE OVERCOME?

One of the most common side effects of a keto diet is bad breath. Not everyone who adopts the keto diet experiences this problem, but it is expected. The difficulty with the breath is due to the processes of internal metabolism. The influence is due to the high metabolization of fats and their conversion into ketone bodies such as acetone. The ketone bodies are broken down into smaller organizations and go into the bloodstream. Then, they enter the lungs through the diffusion process, and eventually, they are expelled through the breath.

You can control breathing difficulties by increasing your water intake. You can also get rid of this problem by practicing good oral hygiene, such as brushing your teeth regularly. Alternatively, you can mask the smell of ketosis by using mints and chewing gum. You should also eat a little more carbohydrate (vegetables) and less protein if you have this problem.

→ DO I NEED ANY SUPPLEMENTS?

By following the keto diet, you may not be getting enough vitamins and minerals your body needs to function normally. Plant-based minerals such as calcium and vitamin D may not be present in your keto diet in the amounts your body requires. Long periods of mineral deficiency can cause a high risk of getting lifestyle diseases such as heart failure.

Heart failure results from the hardening of the heart muscles due to a lack of selenium. Selenium is an essential antioxidant usually found in plant-based foods or nuts (such as Amazonian walnuts). Selenium deficiency is a hardening of your heart muscles that leads to heart failure. To overcome this problem, eat plenty of fruits and vegetables to get vitamins. You can also use beneficial supplements to treat the deficiencies, which come with the keto diet.

Also, you may experience fatigue once you adopt a keto diet. Fatigue is caused by the absence of glucose in the central nervous system. Don't worry! In a few days, this side effect will last, and it may still cause a lot of discomfort and fear on your part. You can easily overcome fatigue by drinking plenty of water and getting enough rest. You can also avoid engaging in strenuous exercises. You can even eat healthy carbohydrates to give you the extra energy your body needs.

→ DOES THE KETO DIET INCREASE THE RISK OF CHRONIC DISEASES, INFLAMMATION, AND OTHERS?

The Keto diet requires you to put a limit on the number of carbohydrates and proteins you consume. When you eat a lot of fat to get enough calories your body needs, you will limit fiber-rich foods such as fruits, legumes, or vegetables. These foods can strengthen your immune system; they are nutrients your body needs to stay healthy. Therefore, limiting your intake of these nutrients increases your risk of chronic diseases such as diabetes, cancer, and high blood pressure. Studies show that chronic diseases can be prevented with diets rich in fruits and vegetables. When you limit their consumption, you reduce their beneficial impact. If you feel this way, eat plenty of fruits and vegetables. You can also incorporate exercise into your keto diet for the best results. Always remember to drink water!

The high-fat consumption required for ketosis can significantly alter cholesterol and lipoproteins' structure; the result is inflammation. This occurs when the cells in your body use a lot of energy to accomplish their normal functioning. Chronic inflammation is also one of the causes of heart disease.

To minimize chronic inflammation, you can control the inflammation problem by eating solid fats and oils. Be sure to also include high-fiber foods in your daily intakes, such as fruits and vegetables.

Keto diets can weaken the immune system in some cases. Dysbiosis is another side effect that can occur when the proper balance of bacteria is altered in your gastrointestinal tract. Highly saturated fats and low levels of fiber in your digestive system are the cause of the disruption. This is especially the case when you ingest diets with little prebiotic fiber. Any impairment of your gastrointestinal tract could damage immune function leading to exposure to chronic disease.

To avoid a weakened immune system, incorporate workouts into your keto diet. You can also eat foods that are high in fiber, such as fruits and vegetables. Also, be sure to drink plenty of water.

A keto diet can also damage your digestive system in the long run. It has been thought that the Keto diet can cause stomach problems such as constipation, high cholesterol levels, diarrhea, kidney stones, and vomiting.

You may also experience abnormal stomach gas. This is normal because the sugar alcohols found in some keto diets can produce gas after digestion. To control gastrointestinal problems, drink plenty of water and eat fiber-rich foods like fruits and vegetables to encourage healthy bacteria's growth in your gastrointestinal system. Get into the habit of exercising regularly.

→ HOW CAN I FACE THE CHALLENGE OF WEIGHT CYCLING?

When you restrict food diets for an extended period, you may gain too much weight when you are not dieting, which you then go on to lose when you are dieting. This process of alternating between weight gain and weight loss is what is called weight cycling. Weight cycling can increase your risk for chronic disease. You can control weight cyclicality by shortening the intervals between diets and the days when you are dieting-free. You should gradually increase the amount of food you consume during free dieting days so that your body has enough time to adjust to the changes in

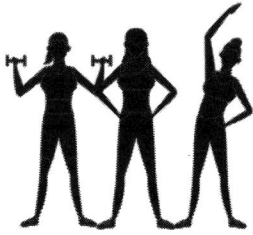

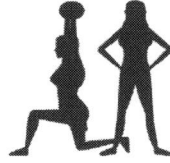

your schedule.

CHAPTER 8: BREAKFAST RECIPES

1. YOGURT WAFFLES

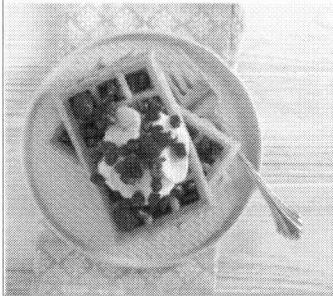

Prep Time: 15 min
Cooking Time: 25 min
Servings: 4
Ingredients:

- ½ cup golden flax seeds meal
- ½ cup plus 3 tbsp. almond flour
- 1½ tbsp. granulated erythritol
- 1 tbsp. unsweetened vanilla whey protein powder
- ½ tsp. organic powder
- ¼ tsp. xanthan gum
- Salt, to taste
- 1 large organic egg, white and yolk separated
- 1 organic whole egg
- 2 tbsp. unsweetened almond milk
- 1½ tbsp. unsalted butter
- 3 oz. plain Greek yogurt
- ¼ tsp. baking soda.

Directions:

1. Preheat the waffle iron and then grease it.
2. In a large bowl, add the flour, erythritol, protein powder, baking soda, baking powder, xanthan gum, salt, and mix until well combined. In a second small bowl, add the egg white and beat until stiff peaks form.
3. In a third bowl, add 2 egg yolks, whole egg, almond milk, butter, yogurt and beat until well combined.
4. Place egg mixture into the bowl of flour mixture and mix until well combined.
5. Gently, fold in the beaten egg whites.
6. Place ¼ cup of the mixture into preheated waffle iron and cook for about 4–5 min. or until golden-brown.
7. Repeat with the remaining mixture.
8. Serve warm.

Nutrition: Calories: 250 kcal Carbs: 3.2 g Total Carbs: 8.8 g Fiber: 5.6 g Sugar: 1.3 g Protein 8.4 g.

2. CHEESE CREPES

Prep Time: 15 min   **Cooking Time:** 20 min   **Servings:** 5

Ingredients:

- 6 ounces cream cheese, softened
- 1/3 cup Parmesan cheese, grated
- 6 large organic eggs
- 1 tsp. granulated Erythritol
- 1½ tbsp. coconut flour
- 1/8 tsp. xanthan gum
- 2 tbsp. unsalted butter

Directions:

1. In a blender, add cream cheese, Parmesan cheese, eggs, and erythritol and pulse on low speed until well combined.
2. While the motor is running, place the coconut flour and xanthan gum and pulse until a thick mixture is formed.
3. Now, pulse on medium speed for a few seconds. Transfer the mixture into a bowl then set aside for about 5 min.
4. Divide the mixture into 10 equal-sized portions. In a nonstick pan, melt butter over medium-low heat. Place 1 portion of

the mixture and tilt the pan to spread into a thin layer.

5. Cook for about 1½ min. or until the edges become brown.

6. Flip the crepe and cook for about 15-20 seconds more. Repeat with the remaining mixture. Serve warm with your favorite keto-friendly filling.

Nutrition: Calories 297 Kcal - Fats 25.1 g - Carbs 3.5 g - Fiber 1.6 g - Proteins 13.7 g

3. BROCCOLI MUFFINS

Prep Time: 15 min   **Cooking Time**: 20 min   **Servings**: 5

Ingredients:

- 2 tbsp. unsalted butter
- 6 large organic eggs
- ½ cup heavy whipping cream
- ½ cup Parmesan cheese, grated
- Salt and ground black pepper, to taste
- 1¼ cup broccoli, chopped
- 2 tbsp. fresh parsley, chopped
- ½ cup Swiss cheese, grated.

Directions:

1. Preheat your oven to 350°F.
2. Grease a 12-cup muffin tin.
3. In a bowl, add the eggs, cream, Parmesan cheese, salt, black pepper and beat until well combined.
4. Divide the broccoli and parsley in the bottom of each prepared muffin cup evenly.
5. Top with the egg mixture, followed by the Swiss cheese.
6. Bake for about 20 min., rotating the pan once halfway through.
7. Remove from the oven and place onto a wire rack for about 5 min. before serving. Carefully, invert the muffins onto a serving platter and serve warm.

Nutrition: Calories: 231 kcal | Total Carbs: 2.5 g | Fiber: 0.5 g | Sugar: 0.9 g | Protein: 13.5 g.

4. RICOTTA PANCAKES

Prep Time.: 10 min   **Cooking Time**: 20 min   **Servings**: 4

Ingredients:

- 4 organic eggs
- ½ cup ricotta cheese
- ¼ cup unsweetened vanilla whey protein powder
- ½ tsp. organic baking powder
- Pinch of salt
- ½ tsp. liquid stevia
- 2 tbsp. unsalted butter

Directions:

1. Using a blender, add all the ingredients and pulse until well combined.
2. In a wok, melt butter over medium heat.
3. Add the desired amount of the mixture and spread it evenly.
4. Cook for about 2–3 min. or until the bottom becomes golden-brown.
5. Flip and cook for about 1–2 min. or until golden brown. Repeat with the remaining mixture. Serve warm.

Nutrition: Calories 184 - Fats 12.9 g - Carbs 2.7 g - Proteins 14.6 g

5. PUMPKIN BREAD

Prep Time: 15 min   **Cooking Time**: 1 h   **Servings**: 5

Ingredients:

- 1⅔ cup almond flour
- 1½ tsp. organic baking powder
- ½ tsp. pumpkin pie spice
- ½ tsp. ground cinnamon
- ½ tsp. ground cloves
- ½ tsp. salt
- 8 oz. cream cheese, softened
- 6 organic eggs, divided
- 1 tbsp. coconut flour
- 1 cup powdered erythritol, divided
- 1 tsp. stevia powder, divided
- 1 tsp. organic lemon extract
- 1 cup homemade pumpkin puree
- ½ cup coconut oil, melted

Directions:

1. Preheat your oven to 325°F.
2. Lightly, grease 2 bread loaf pans.
3. In a bowl, place almond flour, baking powder, spices, salt and mix until well combined.
4. In a second bowl, add the cream cheese, 1 egg, coconut flour, ¼ cup of erythritol, ¼ tsp. of the stevia and with a wire whisk, beat until smooth.
5. In a third bowl, add the pumpkin puree, oil, 5 eggs, ¾ cup of the erythritol, ¾ tsp. of the stevia, and with a wire whisk, beat until well combined. Add the pumpkin mixture into the bowl of the flour mixture and mix until just combined.
6. Place about ¼ of the pumpkin mixture into each loaf pan evenly.
7. Top each pan with the cream cheese mixture evenly, followed by the remaining pumpkin mixture. Bake for about 50–60 min. or until a toothpick inserted in the center comes out clean.
8. Remove the bread pans from oven and place onto a wire rack and let it be for 10 min.
9. With a sharp knife, cut each bread loaf in the desired-sized slices and serve.

Nutrition: Calories: 216 kcal | Total Carbs: 4.5 g | Fiber: 2 g | Sugar: 1.1 g | Protein: 3.4 g.

6. EGGS IN AVOCADO CUPS

Prep.: 10 min **Cooking Time:** 20 min **Servings:** 4

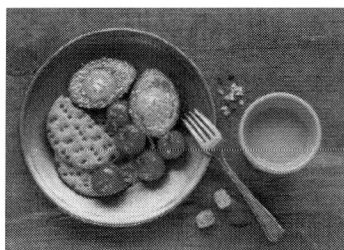

Ingredients:

- 2 ripe avocados, halved and pitted
- 4 organic eggs
- Salt and ground black pepper, as required
- 4 tbsp. cheddar cheese, shredded
- 2 cooked bacon slices, chopped
- 1 tbsp. scallion greens, chopped

Directions:

1. Preheat your oven to 400°F.
2. Carefully, remove abut about 2 tbsp. of flesh from each avocado half. Place avocado halves into a small baking dish.
3. Carefully, crack an egg in each avocado half and sprinkle with salt and black pepper. Top each egg with cheddar cheese evenly.
4. Bake for about 20 min. or until the desired doneness of the eggs.
5. Serve immediately with the garnishing of bacon and chives.

Nutrition: Calories 343 - Fats 29.1 g - Carbs 7.9 g - Fiber 5.7 g - Proteins 13.8 g

7. ARTICHOKE SPINACH BREAKFAST BAKE

Prep Time: 15 min   **Cooking Time:** 20 min   **Servings:** 7

Ingredients:

- ¼ cup milk, fat-free
- ¼ tsp. ground pepper
- ⅓ cup red pepper, diced

- ½ cup feta cheese crumbles
- ½ cup scallions, finely sliced
- ¾ cup canned artichokes, chopped, drained, & patted dry
- 1¼ tsp. kosher salt
- 1 clove garlic, minced
- 1 tbsp. dill, chopped
- 10 oz. spinach, frozen, chopped & drained
- 2 tbsp. parmesan cheese, grated
- 4 large egg whites
- 8 large eggs.

Directions:

1. Preheat the oven to 375°F and grease a large baking dish with nonstick spray or preferred fat source. In a small bowl, combine the spinach, artichoke, scallions, garlic, red pepper, and fill.
2. Combine completely and then pour into the baking dish, spreading into an even layer.
3. In a mixing bowl, combine eggs, egg whites, salt, pepper, parmesan, and milk.
4. Whisk until completely combined, then add feta and mix once more. Pour the egg mixture evenly over the vegetables in the baking dish.
5. Bake for about 35 min., until a butter knife inserted in the center comes out clean.
6. Allow to cool for about 10 min. before cutting into eight equal pieces.
7. Serve warm!

Nutrition: Calories: 574 kcal Carbs: 2 g Fiber: 0.7 g Sugar: 0.1 g Protein: 47 g Fat: 54 g Sodium: 254 mg.

8. CHEDDAR SCRAMBLE

Prep. Time: 10 min.   **Cooking Time**: 8 min.   **Servings**: 6

Ingredients:

- 2 tbsp. olive oil
- 1 small yellow onion, chopped finely
- 12 large organic eggs, beaten lightly
- Salt and ground black pepper, as required
- 4 ounces cheddar cheese, shredded

Directions:

1. In a large wok, heat oil over medium heat and sauté the onion for about 4–5 min.
2. Add the eggs, salt, and black pepper and cook for about 3 min., stirring continuously.
3. Remove from the heat and immediately, stir in the cheese.
4. Serve immediately.

Nutrition: Calories 264 - Fats 20.9 g - Carbs 2.1 g - Fiber 0.3 g - Proteins 17.4 g

9. GRANOLA BARS

Prep Time: 15 min   **Cooking Time**: 20 min   **Servings**: 6

Ingredients:

- 2 cups almonds, chopped
- ½ cup pumpkin seeds, raw
- ⅓ cup coconut flakes, unsweetened
- 2 tbsp. hemp seeds
- ¼ cup clear Sukrin Fiber Syrup
- ¼ cup almond butter
- ¼ cup erythritol, powdered,
- or equal measure of preferred sweetener
- 2 tsp. vanilla extract
- ½ tsp. sea salt.

Directions:

1. Line a small, square baking dish with parchment paper. In a mixing bowl, combine almonds, pumpkin seeds, coconut flakes, and hemp seeds. Stir until evenly mixed.

2. Over medium heat combines the syrup, almond butter, sweetener, salt, and stir until it's smooth and easy to pull the spoon through.

3. Remove the pan from the heat and stir the vanilla extract into the mixture. Pour the syrup over the seeds and stir completely.

4. Pour the mixture into the baking dish and press evenly into one layer and press until the top is even. Let cool completely and slice into 12 bars.

Nutrition: Calories: 254 kcal Carbs: 2 g Sugar: 0.1 g Fiber: 0.7 g Protein: 42.5 g Fat: 47 g Sodium: 145 mg.

10. BACON OMELET

Prep. Time: 10 min.   **Cooking Time**: 15 min.   **Servings**: 2

Ingredients:

- 4 large organic eggs
- 1 tbsp. fresh chives, minced
- Salt and ground black pepper, as required
- 4 bacon slices
- 1 tbsp. unsalted butter
- 2 ounces cheddar cheese, shredded

Directions:

1. In a bowl, add the eggs, chives, salt, and black pepper, and beat until well combined.

2. Heat a non-stick frying pan over medium-high heat and cook the bacon slices for about 8–10 min. To drain place, the bacon onto a paper towel-lined plate. Then chop the bacon slices.

3. With paper towels, wipe out the frying pan.

4. In the same frying pan, melt butter over medium-low heat and cook the egg mixture for about 2 min.

5. Carefully, flip the omelet and top with chopped bacon. Cook for 1–2 min. or until the desired doneness of eggs.

6. Remove from heat and immediately, place the cheese in the center of the omelet.

7. Fold the edges of the omelet over the cheese and cut into 2 portions. Serve immediately.

Nutrition: Calories 427 - Fats 28.2 g - Carbs 1.2 g - Proteins 29.1 g

11. FRENCH TOAST WITH GINGER

Prep Time: 5 min   **Cooking Time**: 10 min   **Servings**: 2

Ingredients:

- 4 whole-wheat bread slices
- ½ cup low-fat milk
- 2 eggs, whisked
- 1 tsp. ground ginger
- Cooking spray.

Directions:

1. Spray the skillet with cooking spray.
2. In the mixing bowl mix up milk and eggs.
3. Then add ginger and dip the bread in the liquid.
4. Roast the bread in the preheated skillet for 2 min. from each side.

Nutrition: Calories: 229 kcal Carbs: 8 g Sugar: 2 g Fiber: 4 g Protein: 29.4 g Fat: 8 g Sodium: 388 mg.

12. PAN EGGS WITH VEGGIES AND PARMESAN

Prep. Time: 5 min.   **Cooking Time**: 15 min.   **Servings**: 6

Ingredients:

- 12 large eggs, whisked
- Salt and pepper
- 1 small red pepper, diced
- 1 small yellow onion, chopped
- 1 cup diced mushrooms
- 1 cup diced zucchini
- 1 cup freshly grated parmesan cheese

Directions:

1. Preheat the oven to 350°F and grease a rimmed baking sheet with cooking spray.
2. Whisk the eggs in a bowl with salt and pepper until frothy. Stir in the peppers, onions, mushrooms, and zucchini until well combined.
3. Pour the mixture into the baking sheet and spread it into an even layer.
4. Sprinkle with parmesan and bake for 12 to 15 min. until the egg is set.
5. Let cool slightly, then cut into squares to serve.

Nutrition: Calories 215 - Fats 14 g - Carbs 5 g - Fiber 1 g - Proteins 18.5 g

13. BAGELS WITH CHEESE

Prep Time: 10 min   **Cooking Time**: 15 min   **Servings**: 6

Ingredients:

- 2½ cup mozzarella cheese
- 1 tsp. baking powder
- 3 oz. cream cheese
- 1½ cup almond flour
- 2 eggs.

Directions:

1. Shred the mozzarella and combine with the flour, baking powder, and cream cheese in a mixing container.
2. Pop into the microwave for about one min. Mix well. Let the mixture cool and add the eggs.
3. Break apart into six sections and shape into round bagels.
4. Note: You can also sprinkle with a seasoning of your choice or pinch of salt if desired.
5. Bake them for approximately 12 to 15 min. Serve or cool and store.

Nutrition: Calories: 374 kcal Carbs: 8 g Protein: 19 g Fats: 31 g.

14. ALMOND BUTTER MUFFINS

Prep. Time: 10 min.   **Cooking Time**: 25 min.   **Servings**: 12

Ingredients:

- 2 cups almond flour
- 1 cup powdered erythritol
- 2 tsp.s baking powder
- ¼ tsp. salt
- ¾ cup almond butter, warmed
- ¾ cup unsweetened almond milk
- 4 large eggs

Directions:

1. Preheat the oven to 350°F and line a muffin pan with paper liners. Whisk the almond flour together with the erythritol, baking powder, and salt in a mixing bowl.
2. In a separate bowl, whisk together the almond milk, almond butter, and eggs.
3. Stir the wet ingredients into the dry until just combined. Spoon the batter into the prepared pan and bake for 22 to 25 min. until a knife inserted in the center comes out clean.
4. Cool the muffins in the pan for 5 min. then turn out them onto a wire cooling rack.

Nutrition: Calories 135 - Fats 11 g - Carbs 4 g - Fiber 2 g - Proteins 6 g

15. BAKED APPLES

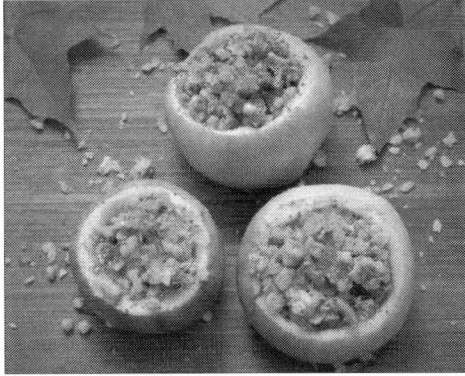

Prep Time: 10 min   **Cooking Time:** 1 h   **Servings:** 4

Ingredients:

- 4 tsp. or to taste Keto-friendly sweetener
- ¾ tsp. cinnamon
- ¼ cup chopped pecans
- 4 large granny Smith apples.

Nutrition: Calories: 175 kcal

Carbs: 16 g

Protein: 6.8 g

Fats: 19.9 g.

Directions:

1. Set the oven temperature at 375°F. Mix the sweetener with the cinnamon and pecans.
2. Core the apple and add the prepared stuffing.
3. Add enough water into the baking dish to cover the bottom of the apple.
4. Bake them for about 45 min. to 1 hour.

16. CLASSIC WESTERN OMELET

Prep. Time: 5 min.   **Cooking Time:** 10 min.   **Servings:** 1

Ingredients:

- 2 tbps coconut oil
- 3 large eggs, whisked
- 1 tbsp. heavy cream
- Salt and pepper
- ¼ cup diced green pepper
- ¼ cup diced yellow onion
- ¼ cup diced ham

Directions:

1. Whisk together the eggs, heavy cream, salt and pepper in a small bowl. Heat 1 tsp. coconut oil in a small skillet over medium heat.
2. Add the peppers, onions, and ham then sauté for 3 to 4 min.
3. Spoon the mixture into a bowl and reheat the skillet with the rest of the oil.
4. Pour in the whisked eggs and cook until the bottom of the egg starts to set.
5. Tilt the pan to spread the egg and cook until almost set. Spoon the veggie and ham mixture over half the omelet and fold it over
6. Let the omelet cook until the eggs are set then serve hot.

Nutrition: Calories 415 - Fats 32.5 g - Carbs 6.5 g - Fiber 1.5 g - Proteins 25 g

17. OMELET WITH PEPPERS

Prep Time: 10 min   **Cooking Time:** 15 min   **Servings:** 4

Ingredients:

- 4 eggs, beaten
- 1 tbsp. margarine
- 1 cup bell peppers, chopped
- 2 oz. scallions, chopped.

Directions:

1. Toss the margarine in the skillet and melt it.
2. In the mixing bowl mix up eggs and bell peppers. Add scallions.
3. Pour the egg mixture in the hot skillet and roast the omelet for 12 min.

Nutrition: Calories: 102 kcal Carbs: 7.3 g Sugar: 3 g Fiber: 0.8 g Fat: 10.8 g Sodium: 98 mg Protein: 6.1 g.

18. SHEET PAN EGGS WITH HAM AND PEPPER JACK

Prep. Time: 5 min.   **Cooking Time:** 15 min.   **Servings:** 6

Ingredients:

- 12 large eggs, whisked
- Salt and pepper
- 2 cups diced ham
- 1 cup shredded pepper jack cheese

Directions:

1. Preheat the oven to 350°F and grease a rimmed baking sheet with cooking spray.
2. Whisk the eggs in a bowl with salt and pepper until frothy. Stir in the ham and cheese until well combined.
3. Pour the mixture into the baking sheet and spread it into an even layer.
4. Bake for 12 to 15 min. until the egg is set. Let cool slightly then cut into squares to serve.

Nutrition: Calories 235 g - Fats 15 g - Carbs 2.5 g - Fiber 0.5 g - Proteins 21 g

---

19. BACON AND SALSA MUFFINS

Prep Time: 10 min.   **Cooking Time:** 30 min.   **Servings:** 8

Ingredients:

- 4 slices bacon, cooked and chopped
- 4 eggs, beaten
- ½ cup almond flour
- ½ cup salsa

Special Equipment:

- 8 muffin cups, greased with olive oil

Directions:

1. Start by preheating the oven to 350°F (180°C).
2. Combine the chopped bacon, beaten eggs, almond flour, and salsa in a bowl. Stir to combine well.
3. Divide and pour the mixture into the muffin cups, then arrange them in the preheated oven.
4. Bake for 30 min. or until the center is springy and a toothpick inserted into the muffin comes out dry.
5. Remove them from the oven and allow to cool for a few min. before serving.
6. To make this a complete meal, serve it with coconut milk or plain Greek yogurt.

Nutrition: Calories: 110 Total Fat: 8.6g Carbs: 2.5g Protein: 5.7g Cholesterol: 99mg Sodium: 237mg

---

20. CRISPY CHAI WAFFLES

Prep. Time: 10 Min   **Cooking Time:** 20 Min.   **Servings:** 4

Ingredients:

- 4 large eggs, separated into whites and yolks
- 3 tbsp. coconut flour
- 3 tbsp. powdered erythritol
- 1 ¼ tsp. baking powder
- 1 tsp. vanilla extract
- ½ tsp. ground cinnamon
- ¼ tsp. ground ginger
- Pinch ground cloves
- Pinch ground cardamom
- 3 tbsp. coconut oil, melted
- 3 tbsp. unsweetened almond milk

Directions:

1. Separate the eggs into two different mixing bowls. Whip the egg whites until stiff peaks form then set aside.
2. Whisk the egg yolks with coconut flour, erythritol, baking powder, vanilla, cinnamon, cardamom, and cloves in the other bowl.
3. Add the melted coconut oil to the second bowl while whisking then whisk in the almond milk.
4. Gently fold in the egg whites until just combined. Now, preheat the waffle iron and grease with cooking spray.
5. Spoon about ½ cup of batter into the iron.
6. Cook the waffle according to the manufacturer's instructions.
7. Remove the waffle to a plate and repeat with the remaining batter.

21. CRUSTLESS FRENCH SPINACH QUICHE

Prep Time: 20 Min.   **Cooking Time:** 30 Min.   **Servings:** 6

Ingredients:

- 1 (10 ounces / 284 g) package frozen chopped spinach, thawed and drained
- 1 tbsp. olive oil
- 1 onion, chopped
- 3 cups Muenster cheese, shredded
- 5 eggs, beaten
- ¼ tsp. salt
- ⅛ tsp. ground black pepper
- 1 tbsp. coconut oil

Directions:

1. Start by preheating the oven to 350ºF (180ºC).
2. Bring a pot of water to a boil. Blanch the spinach in the water for 10 seconds to reduce the concentration of the oxalic acid. Set aside.
3. Drizzle the olive oil into a nonstick skillet and warm over medium-high heat, then sauté the onions in the skillet for 5 min. or until translucent. Add the blanched spinach and sauté for 3 to 4 min. or until wilted.
4. Transfer the sautéed spinach and onions to a large bowl, then add the shredded Muenster cheese, beaten eggs, salt, and ground black pepper. Blend well to combine.
5. Drizzle a pie pan with coconut oil. Gently pour the mixture into the pan.
6. Arrange the pan into the preheated oven and cook for 30 min. until cooked through. Remove the pan from the oven and allow to cool for a few min., then slice to serve.
7. To make this a complete meal, serve the omelet on a bed of greens. They also taste great paired with roast beef sirloin.

Nutrition: Calories: 309 | Total Fat: 24.1g | Carbs: 4.8g | Protein: 19.8g | Cholesterol: 209mg | Sodium: 546mg

22. BACON CHEESEBURGER WAFFLES

Prep. Time: 10 Min.   **Cooking:** 20 Min.   **Servings:** 4

Ingredients:

Toppings:
- Pepper and Salt to taste
- 1.5 ounces of cheddar cheese
- 4 tbsp. of sugar-free barbecue sauce
- 4 slices of bacon
- 4 ounces of ground beef, 70% lean meat and 30% fat

Waffle dough:

- Pepper and salt to taste
- 3 tbsp. of parmesan cheese, grated
- 4 tbsp. of almond flour
- ¼ tsp. of onion powder
- ¼ tsp. of garlic powder
- 1 cup (125 g) of cauliflower crumbles
- 2 large eggs
- 1.5 ounces of cheddar cheese

Directions:

1. Shred about 3 ounces of cheddar cheese then add in cauliflower crumbles in a bowl and put in half of the cheddar cheese.
2. Put into the mixture spices, almond flour, eggs and parmesan cheese then mix and put aside for some time.
3. Thinly slice the bacon and cook in a skillet on medium to high heat.
4. After the bacon is cooked partially, put in the beef. Cook until the mixture is well done.
5. Then put the excess grease from the bacon mixture into the waffle mixture. Set aside the bacon mix.
6. Use an immersion blender to blend the waffle mix until it becomes a paste then add into the waffle iron half of the mix and cook until it becomes crispy.

7. Repeat for the remaining waffle mixture.
8. As the waffles cook, add sugar-free barbecue sauce to the ground beef and bacon mixture in the skillet.
9. Then proceed to assemble waffles by topping them with half of the left cheddar cheese and half the beef mixture. 10. Repeat this for the remaining waffles, broil for around 1-2 min. until the cheese has melted then serve right away.

Nutrition: Calories 405 - Fats 33 g - Carbs 4.5 - Fiber 1.4 - Proteins 18.8 g

23. EASY BAKED KETO BREAD

Prep Time: 15 Min.   **Cooking Time**: 45 Min.   **Servings** 12

Ingredients:

- 7 eggs, beaten
- ½ cup butter, melted
- 2 tbsp. olive oil
- 2 cups blanched almond flour
- ½ tsp. xanthan gum
- 1 tsp. baking powder
- ½ tsp. sea salt

Directions:

1. Start by preheating the oven to 350ºF (180ºC).
2. Make the bread: Combine the beaten eggs with butter and olive oil in a large bowl. Mix the almond flour, xanthan gum, baking powder, and salt together in a separate bowl. Pour the dry mixture into the egg mixture gently. Keep stirring until it has a thick consistency.
3. Pour the mixture into a lightly greased baking pan. Press the mixture with a spatula so it covers the bottom evenly.
4. Arrange the pan into the preheated oven and bake for 45 min. or until crisp and lightly browned.
5. Remove the bread from the oven. Allow to cool for a few min. before serving.
6. To make this a complete meal, you can use the keto bread to serve as a part of sandwich or hamburger, or you can serve it with coconut milk and fried eggs.

Nutrition: Calories: 247 Total Fat: 22.1g Carbs: 4.9g Protein: 7.7g Cholesterol: 116mg Sodium: 209mg

24. KETO BREAKFAST CHEESECAKE

Prep. Time: 20 Min.   **Cooking:** 45 Min.   **Servings:** 24

Ingredients:

Toppings:
- 1/4 cup of mixed berries for each cheesecake thawed

Filling:
- ½ tsp. of vanilla extract
- ½ tsp. of almond extract
- 3/4 cup of sweetener

- 6 eggs
- 8 ounces of cream cheese
- 16 ounces of cottage cheese

Crust:
- 4 tbsp. of salted butter
- 2 tbsp. of sweetener
- 2 cups of almonds, whole

Directions:

1. Preheat oven to around 350°F.
2. Pulse almonds in a food processor then add in butter and sweetener. Pulse until all the ingredients mix well.
3. Coat twelve silicone muffin pans using foil or paper liners.
4. Divide the batter evenly between the muffin pans then press into the bottom part until it forms a crust and bakes for about 8 min.
5. In the meantime, mix in a food processor

the cream cheese and cottage cheese then pulse until the mixture is smooth.

6. Put in the extracts and sweetener then combine until well mixed.

7. Add in eggs and pulse again until it becomes smooth; you might need to scrape down the mixture from the sides of the processor. Share equally the batter

between the muffin pans, then bake for around 30-40 min. until the middle is not wobbly when you shake the muffin pan lightly.

8. Put aside until cooled completely then put in the refrigerator for about 2 hours and then top with thawed berries.

Nutrition: Calories 152 - Fats 12 g - Carbs 3 g - Fiber 0.5 g - Proteins 6 g

25. FRENCH CREPES

Prep Time: 10 Min.   **Cooking Time**: 20 Min.   **Servings** 4

Ingredients:

- 2 eggs, beaten
- ¼ cup coconut flour
- ½ cup coconut milk
- ½ cup water
- 2 tbsp. butter, melted
- ¼ tsp. salt

Directions:

1. Combine the beaten eggs with coconut flour in a large bowl. Pour into the coconut milk and water slowly and gradually and keep stirring. Then fold in the butter and salt. Blend the mixture until smooth.

2. Make a crepe: Warm a greased frying pan over medium-high heat, then spoon ¼ cup of the

mixture into the pan and swirl the pan so the mixture covers the bottom evenly.

3. Cook for 4 min., flipping the crepe halfway through or until golden brown. Then transfer the cooked crepe to a serving dish and slice to serve.

4. To make it a complete meal, you can serve the crepes with sugar-free strawberry syrup.

Nutrition: Calories: 187 Total Fat: 17.6g Carbs: 2.7g Protein: 5.3g Cholesterol: 325mg Sodium: 263mg

26. KETO EGG-CRUST PIZZA

Prep. Time: 5 Min.   **Cooking**: 15 Min.   **Servings**: 1-2

Ingredients:

- ¼ tsp. of dried oregano to taste
- ½ tsp. of spike seasoning to taste
- 1 ounce of mozzarella, chopped into small cubes
- 6 – 8 sliced thinly black olives
- 6 slices of turkey pepperoni, sliced into half
- 4-5 thinly sliced small grape tomatoes
- 2 eggs, beaten well
- 1-2 tsp.s of olive oil

Directions:

1. Preheat the broiler in an oven than in a small bowl, beat well the eggs.

2. Cut the pepperoni and tomatoes into slices then cut the mozzarella cheese into cubes.

3. Put some olive oil in a skillet over medium heat than heat the pan for around one min. until it begins to get hot.

4. Add in eggs and season with oregano and spike seasoning then cook for around 2 min. until the eggs begin to set at the bottom.

5. Drizzle half of the mozzarella, olives, pepperoni and tomatoes on the eggs followed

by another layer of the remaining half of the above ingredients.

6. Ensure that there is a lot of cheese on the topmost layers.

7. Cover the skillet using a lid and cook until the cheese begins to melt, and the eggs are set, for around 3-4 min.

8. Place the pan under the preheated broiler, cook until the top gets brown color, and the cheese has melted nicely for around 2-3 min.

9. Serve immediately.

Nutrition: Calories 363 - Fats 24 g - Carbs 20.8 g - Fiber 1.2 g - Proteins 19.2 g

27. MEDITERRANEAN SHAKSHUKA

Prep Time: 20 Min.   **Cooking Time**: 20 Min.   **Servings** 4

Ingredients:

- 2 cups tomatoes, chopped
- 1 hot chile pepper, seeded and finely chopped, or to taste
- 1 tsp. paprika
- 1 tsp. ground cumin
- 1 tsp. salt
- 3 tbsp. olive oil
- 1 cup bell peppers, thinly sliced
- 1⅓ cups onion, chopped
- 2 cloves garlic, minced, or to taste
- 4 eggs

Directions:

1. Mix the tomatoes, hot chile pepper, paprika, cumin, and salt in a medium bowl. Set aside.
2. Drizzle the olive in a nonstick skillet and heat over medium heat, then add the bell peppers, onion, and garlic. Sauté for 5 min. or until the onion is translucent and the peppers are wilted. Pour the tomato mixture into the skillet. Stir to mix well. Let them simmer for 10 min. or until the tomato juice evaporates.
3. Make four wells in the mixture and break each egg into each well. Cover the skillet with lid and cook for 5 min. until firm.
4. Turn off the heat and allow them to cool for a few min. before serving.
5. Sprinkle with minced green onion will bring the recipe a fresher taste.

Nutrition: Calories: 209 Total Fat: 16g Carbs: 10.5g Protein: 5.2g Cholesterol: 164mg Sodium: 654mg

28. BREAKFAST ROLL-UPS

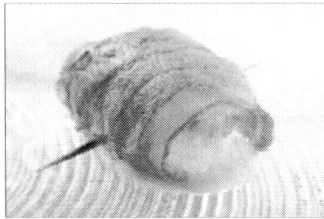

Prep. Time: 5 Min. **Cooking**: 15 Min. **Servings**: 5 Roll-Ups

Ingredients:

- Non-stick cooking spray
- 5 patties of cooked breakfast sausage
- 5 slices of cooked bacon
- 1.5 cups of cheddar cheese, shredded
- Pepper and salt
- 10 large eggs

Directions:

1. Preheat a skillet on medium to high heat then using a whisk, combine two of the eggs in a mixing bowl.
2. After the pan has become hot, lower the heat to medium-low heat then put in the eggs. If you want to, you can utilize some cooking spray.
3. Season eggs with some pepper and salt.
4. Cover the eggs and leave them to cook for a couple of min.
5. Drizzle around 1/3 cup of cheese on top of the eggs then place a strip of bacon and divide the sausage into two and place on top.
6. Roll the eggs carefully on top of the fillings. The roll-up will almost look like a taquito. If you have a hard time folding over the eggs, use a spatula to keep them intact until they have molded into a roll-up. Put aside the roll-up then repeat the above steps until you have four more roll-ups; you should have 5 roll-ups in total.

Nutrition: Calories 412 - Fats 31.6 g - Carbs 2.2 g - Fiber 1.3 g - Proteins 28.2 g

29. EGG FOO YOUNG

Prep Time: 45 min.   **Cooking Time**: 2 min   **Servings**: 10 patties

Ingredients:

- 6 Large Eggs
- 1/4 Cup Coconut Flour
- Kosher Salt, To Taste

- 1/2 Tsp. Apple Cider Vinegar
- 1 Cup Ham, Cooked & Diced
- 1 & 1/4 Cups Spinach, Frozen
- 2 Scallions, Sliced
- 1 Tbsp. Cilantro Fresh & Minced
- 1/2 Tsp. Baking Soda
- Black Pepper, Freshly Ground
- Avocado Oil

Directions:

1. Take a bowl and combine the coconut flour, eggs, apple cider vinegar, and salt together with a whisk to make a smooth mixture.
2. Add in the thawed spinach, cilantro, scallions, ham, black pepper, and baking soda. Mix them well.
3. Heat avocado oil in a non-stick frying pan and spread a spoonful of batter in it with the back of the spoon. Do not turn the side for 2 min. at medium heat and cook both sides well.
4. Once done, take out in a dish and repeat the process until the batter is finished.

Nutrients: Calories: 124 kcal Fat: 9g Carbohydrates: 3g Protein: 7g Fiber: 2g

30. TACO BOWLS

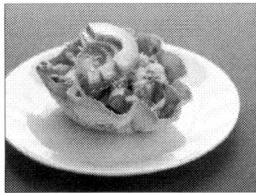

Prep. Time: 35 min.   **Cooking Time:** 5 min   **Servings**: 6

Ingredients:

Cauli Rice:
- 1 & 1/2 Cups Cauliflower Rice
- 6 Large Eggs, Beaten
- 3 Tbsps. Avocado Oil

- 2 Cups Ground Beef
- 1 Jalapeño Pepper, Minced
- 2 Tbsps. Lime Juice
- 2 Tbsps. Broth Or Water
- 1 Tsp. Onion Powder
- 2 Tsps. Taco Seasoning
- 2 Tsps. Milk, Dairy-Free
- Sea Salt, To Taste
- Black Pepper, To Taste
- Additional Toppings:
- Fresh Salsa
- 1 Cup Cherry Tomatoes, Halved
- 1 Avocado, Sliced
- Cilantro, Minced
- Lime Juice, To Taste

Directions:

1. Heat one tbsp. avocado oil in a skillet and stir fry the cauliflower rice in it over medium flame. Let it cook for about 2-3 min., covered.
2. Then stir again and add in the lime juice, minced jalapeño, salt, and pepper. Mix until the required texture is attained. Remove from the heat and dish out. Set aside.
3. Put one tbsp. avocado oil in the same skillet and brown the ground beef in it over medium-high flame. Add the onion powder, salt, and taco seasoning in it and stir well to combine.
4. Reduce the flame to medium-low and add the broth or water to it. Stir for a few min. until cooked thoroughly and remove from the heat. Take a bowl and whisk the eggs in it with milk and some salt and pepper.
5. Heat one tbsp. of avocado oil in a pan over medium flame and pour the whisked eggs in it. Cook and stir the eggs to scramble them. Once cooked, remove from the heat.
6. Take serving bowls and put layers of cauliflower rice, seasoned beef, scrambled eggs, and additional toppings.

Nutrients: Calories: 413 kcal Fat: 33g Carbohydrates: 8g Protein: 22g Fiber: 4g

31. CHAFFLES

Prep. Time: 10 min.   **Cooking Time**: 3 min.   **Servings**: 4

Ingredients:
- 2 Eggs
- 1 Cup Mozzarella Cheese, Finely Shredded
- Cooking Spray

Directions:

1. Preheat waffle iron and spray it with cooking spray.

2. Take a bowl and put egg and cheese in it. Whisk it well.
3. Pour one-quarter of the mixture on the preheated waffle iron and let it cook until golden brown, for about 2 to 3 min.
4. Repeat the same for the remaining batter.
5. You can use chaffles as sandwich bread or eat with maple syrup as it is.

Nutrients: Calories: 115 kcal Fat: 8g Carbohydrates: 1g Protein: 9g Sugar: 2g

32. PULLED PORK BREAKFAST HASH

Prep. Time: 20 min.   **Cooking Time**: 5 min.   **Servings**: 4

Ingredients:

- 2 Eggs
- 2 Tbsps. Olive Oil
- 1/4 Tsp. Garlic Powder
- 1/3 Cup Pulled Pork
- 3 Brussels Sprouts, Halved
- 1/4 Tsp. Black Pepper
- 1 Cup Spinach, Chopped
- 1 Turnip, Diced
- 1/2 Tsp. Paprika
- 2 Tbsps. Red Onion, Diced
- 1/4 Tsp. Salt
- 1 Tbsp. Parsley, Finely Chopped

Directions:

1. Take a skillet and heat olive oil in it. Sauté the diced onion with all the spices in it for about 5 min., over medium-high flame. Next, add in the other vegetables and cook for a few more min. until they become soft.
2. Put the pulled pork in it as well and stir fry it. Crack two eggs on it and cover it.
3. Let it cook until the egg whites are not runny anymore, for about 4-5 min.
4. Top with chopped parsley.

Nutrients: Calories: 153 kcal Fat: 10g Carbohydrates: 8g Protein: 6g Fiber: 1g

33. PARMESAN CHEESE AND BABY SPINACH OMELET

Prep Time: 6 Min.   **Cooking Time**: 9 Min.   **Servings**: 1

Ingredients:

- 1½ tbsp. Parmesan cheese, grated
- 1 cup baby spinach leaves, torn
- 2 eggs
- ⅛ tsp. ground nutmeg
- ¼ tsp. onion powder
- Salt and ground black pepper, to taste
- 1 tbsp. olive oil

Directions:

1. Whisk the eggs in a large bowl, then mix in the grated Parmesan cheese and spinach. Sprinkle the nutmeg, onion powder, salt, and ground black pepper to season.
2. Make the omelet: Drizzle a nonstick skillet with olive oil and heat over medium heat. Pour in the mixture and cook for 6 min., flipping the omelet halfway through the cooking time.
3. Lower the heat and cook for 2 or 3 min. more until the omelet reaches your desired doneness.
4. Top the cooked omelet with ketchup, if desired, and slice to serve.
5. To make it a complete meal, you can serve the omelet with seasoned bacon rolls and avocado wedges.

Nutrients: Calories: 301 Total Fat: 21.6g Carbs: 4.8g Protein: 21g Cholesterol: 1244mg Sodium: 367mg

34. MUSHROOM AND OLIVE OMELET

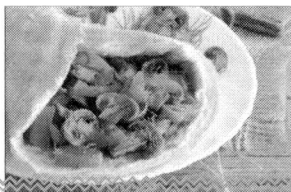

Prep Time: 15 Min.   **Cooking Time**: 30 Min. **Servings**: 8

Ingredients:

- 1 (12 ounces / 340 g) can mushrooms, sliced
- 1 (6 ounces / 170 g) can black olives, sliced
- 12 eggs, scrambled
- ¼ cup butter
- 1 small onion, chopped
- ½ cup coconut milk
- ½ tsp. salt
- ½ tsp. ground black pepper
- 1½ cups Cheddar cheese, shredded
- Cooked ham, chopped (optional)
- Jalapeño peppers, sliced (optional)

Directions:

1. Start by preheating the oven to 400°F (205°C).
2. Put the butter in a nonstick skillet and melt over medium heat. Swirl the skillet so the butter covers the bottom evenly. Add the chopped onion and sauté for 5 to 7 min. or until translucent. Let it stand for later use.
3. Combine the scrambled eggs with coconut milk in a large bowl, then sprinkle with salt and ground black pepper. Stir to mix well. Set aside.
4. Make the omelet: Put the shredded Cheddar cheese in a greased baking pan, then top the cheese with sautéed onion, ham, mushrooms, olives, and jalapeño, and then pour over the egg mixture. Arrange the baking pan into the preheated oven without stirring the mixture. Bake for 30 min., flipping the omelet halfway through the cooking time. To check the doneness, cut a small slit in the center of the omelet, if raw eggs run into the cut, bake for another few min.
5. Remove the baked omelet from the oven. Let it sit for a few min. and slice to serve.
6. To make it a complete meal, you can serve the omelet with seasoned bacon rolls and avocado wedges.

Nutrients: Calories: 344 Total Fat: 27.3g Carbs: 7.2g Protein: 17.9g Cholesterol: 254mg Sodium: 1087mg

35. VEGGIES AND SAUSAGE FRITTATA

Prep Time: 10 Min.　　**Cooking Time**: 30 Min.　**Servings**: 6

Ingredients:

- 8 eggs
- 8 drops hot pepper sauce, or more to taste
- 2 tbsp. heavy cream
- 4 ounces (113 g) bulk breakfast sausage, crumbled
- 2 tbsp. butter
- ⅔ cup red bell pepper, chopped
- ½ cup onion, chopped
- 1 cup mushrooms, chopped
- Salt and ground black pepper, to taste
- ½ cup chopped fresh spinach, blanched
- 1 cup Cheddar cheese, shredded

Directions:

1. Start by preheating the oven to 325°F (160°C).
2. Whisk together the eggs, hot pepper sauce, and heavy cream. Set aside. To make the frittata, sauté the sausage in a nonstick skillet over medium heat for 4 min., then add and melt the butter. Swirl the skillet so the butter coats the bottom evenly.
4. Put in the red bell pepper, onion, mushrooms, salt, and ground black pepper and sauté for 4 min. until the onion is translucent.
5. Add the spinach and sauté for 1 min. Remove the mixture from the skillet to a baking pan. Sprinkle the cheese on top and pour over the egg mixture.
6. Arrange the pan into the preheated oven and bake for 20 min. You can check the doneness by cutting a slit in the center of the frittata, if raw eggs run into the cut, then baking for another few min.
7. Remove the baking pan from the oven. Allow to cool for a few min., and slice to serve.
8. To make this a complete meal, you can serve the omelet with cherry tomatoes and beef steak.

Nutrients: Calories: 283 Total Fat: 22.7g Carbs: 3.8g Protein: 16.5g Cholesterol: 295mg Sodium: 443mg

36. BREAKFAST WITH SAUSAGE CASSEROLE

Prep Time: 15 Min.　　**Cooking Time**: 21 Min.　**Servings**: 4

Ingredients:

- 1.5 pounds (680 g) pork sausage, crumbled
- 1 (8 ounces / 227 g) package gluten-free crescent roll
- 4 eggs, beaten
- 2 cups mozzarella cheese, shredded
- ¾ cup coconut milk
- Salt and ground black pepper, to taste

Directions:

1. Start by preheating the oven to 425°F (220°C).
2. Cook the sausage in a nonstick skillet over medium heat for 6 min. until browned. Transfer the cooked sausage into a large bowl.
3. Add the beaten eggs, mozzarella cheese, coconut milk, salt, and ground black pepper to the bowl. Stir to combine well. Set aside.
4. Flatten the crescent rolls on a clean working surface with a rolling pin. Lay the flattened crescent rolls on a greased casserole dish.
5. Pour the sausage mixture over the crescent rolls. Arrange the casserole dish into the preheated oven and bake for 15 min. You can check the doneness by cutting a small slit in the center, if raw eggs run into the cut, then baking for another few min.
6. Remove the casserole dish from the oven and allow it to cool before serving.

Nutrients: Calories: 389 Total Fat: 31.8g Carbs: 9.3 Protein: 15.1g Cholesterol: 114mg Sodium: 671mg

37. SCRAMBLED EGG AND SAUSAGE MUFFINS

Prep Time: 10 Min.　　**Cooking Time**: 20 Min.　**Servings**: 12

Ingredients:

- 12 eggs
- 8 ounces (227 g) bulk pork sausage, crumbled
- 2 tbsp. olive oil
- ½ cup onion, chopped
- ½ cup chopped green bell pepper, or to taste
- ½ cup Cheddar cheese, shredded
- ¼ tsp. garlic powder
- ½ tsp. salt
- ¼ tsp. ground black pepper

SPECIAL EQUIPMENT:

- 12 muffin cups, greased with olive oil

Directions:

1. Start by preheating the oven to 350°F (180°C).
2. Warm a nonstick skillet over medium heat. Put in the sausage and sauté for 10 min. or until well browned. Remove from the skillet and set aside.
3. Clean the skillet and drizzle with olive oil. Add the chopped onion into the skillet and sauté for 3 min. or until the onion is half translucent, then break the eggs into the skillet and sauté for 3 min. or until the eggs are scrambled, and then add the green bell pepper, shredded cheese, garlic powder, salt, and ground black pepper and cook for 2 min. more until the cheese melts.
4. Fold in the cooked sausage and sauté to combine. Spoon ⅓ cup of the mixture in a muffin cup. Repeat with the remaining mixture and muffin cups. Arrange the muffin cups in the preheated oven.
5. Bake for 20 min. or until the tops of the muffins spring back when gently pressed with your fingers.
6. Remove from the oven. Allow to cool for a few min. before serving.
7. You can arrange the muffins over a green bed to serve and sprinkle with Italian seasoning (without salt and black pepper).

Nutrients: Calories: 196 Total Fat: 14.9g Carbs: 2.1g Protein: 12.7g Cholesterol: 202mg Sodium: 365mg

38. FROZEN KETO COFFEE

Prep. Time: 5 Min　　**Cooking Time**: 20 Min　**Servings**: 1

Ingredients:

- 12 ounces coffee, chilled
- 1 scoop MCT powder (or 1 tbsp. MCT oil)
- 1 tbsp. heavy (whipping) cream
- Pinch ground cinnamon
- Dash sweetener (optional)
- ½ cup ice

Directions:
1. In a blender, combine the coffee, MCT powder, cream, cinnamon, sweetener (if using), and ice.
2. Blend until smooth.

Nutrition: Calories 127 - Fats 13 g - Carbs 1.5 g - Fiber 1 g - Proteins 1 g

39. NO-BAKE KETO POWER BARS

Prep. Time: 10 Min.   **Cooking Time**: 0 Min.   **Servings**: 12 Bars

Ingredients:
- ½ cup pili nuts
- ½ cup whole hazelnuts
- ½ cup walnut halves
- ¼ cup hulled sunflower seeds
- ¼ cup unsweetened coconut flakes or chips
- ¼ cup hulled hemp seeds
- 2 tbsp. unsweetened cacao nibs
- 2 scoops of collagen powder (I use 1 scoop Perfect Keto vanilla collagen and 1 scoop Perfect Keto unflavored collagen powder)
- ½ tsp. ground cinnamon
- ½ tsp. sea salt
- ¼ cup coconut oil, melted
- 1 tsp. vanilla extract
- Stevia or monk fruit to sweeten (optional if you are using unflavored collagen powder)

Directions:
1. Line a 9-inch square baking pan with parchment paper.
2. In a food processor or blender, combine the pili nuts, hazelnuts, walnuts, sunflower seeds, coconut, hemp seeds, cacao nibs, collagen powder, cinnamon, and salt and pulse a few times.
3. Add the coconut oil, vanilla extract, and sweetener (if using). Pulse again until the ingredients are combined. Do not over-pulse or it will turn to mush. You want the nuts and seeds to have some texture still.
4. Pour the mixture into the prepared pan and press it into an even layer. Cover with another piece of parchment (or fold over extra from the first piece) and place a heavy pot or dish on top to help press the bars together.
5. Refrigerate overnight and then cut into 12 bars. Store the bars in individual storage bags in the refrigerator for a quick grab-and-go breakfast.

Nutrition: Calories 242 - Fats 22 g - Carbs 4.5 g - Fiber 2.5 g - Proteins 6.5 g

40. EASY SKILLET PANCAKES

Prep. Time: 5 Min.   **Cooking Time**: 5 Min.   **Servings**: 8

Ingredients:
1. 8 ounces cream cheese
2. 8 eggs
3. 2 tbsp. coconut flour
4. 2 tsps baking powder
5. 1 tsp. ground cinnamon
6. ½ tsp. vanilla extract
7. 1 tsp. liquid stevia or sweetener of choice (optional)
8. 2 tbsp. butter

Directions:
1. In a blender, combine the cream cheese, eggs, coconut flour, baking powder, cinnamon, vanilla, and stevia (if using). Blend until smooth. In a large skillet over medium heat, melt the butter.
2. Use half the mixture to pour four evenly sized pancakes and cook for about a min., until you see bubbles on top. Flip the pancakes and cook for another min. Remove from the pan and add more

butter or oil to the skillet if needed. Repeat with the remaining batter.
3. Top with butter and eat right away or freeze the pancakes in a freezer-safe

resealable bag with sheets of parchment in between, for up to 1 month.

Nutrition: Calories 179 - Fats 15 g - Carbs 3 g - Fiber 1 g - Proteins 8 g

41. QUICK KETO BLENDER MUFFINS

Prep. Time: 5 Min. **Cooking Time**: 25 Min. **Servings**: 12

Ingredients:

- Butter, ghee, or coconut oil for greasing the pan
- 6 eggs
- 8 ounces cream cheese, at room temperature
- 2 scoops flavored collagen powder
- 1 tsp. ground cinnamon
- 1 tsp. baking powder
- Few drops or dash sweetener (optional)

Directions:

1. Preheat the oven to 350°F. Grease a 12-cup muffin pan very well with butter, ghee, or coconut oil.
2. Alternatively, you can use silicone cups or paper muffin liners.
3. In a blender, combine the eggs, cream cheese, collagen powder, cinnamon, baking powder, and sweetener (if using).
4. Blend until well combined and pour the mixture into the muffin cups, dividing equally.
5. Bake for 22 to 25 min. until the muffins are golden brown on top and firm.
6. Let cool then store in a glass container or plastic bag in the refrigerator for up to 2 weeks or in the freezer for up to 3 months.
7. To servings refrigerated muffins, heat in the microwave for 30 seconds.
8. To meals from frozen, thaw in the refrigerator overnight and then microwave for 30 seconds, or microwave straight from the freezer for 45 to 60 seconds or until heated through.

Nutrition: Calories 120 - Fats 10 g - Carbs 1.5 g - Proteins 6 g

42. KETO EVERYTHING BAGELS

Prep. Time: 10 min. **Cooking time**: 15 min. **Servings**: 8

Ingredients:

- 2 cups shredded mozzarella cheese
- 2 tbsp. labneh cheese (or cream cheese)
- 1½ cups almond flour
- 1 egg
- 2 tsp.s baking powder
- ¼ tsp. sea salt
- 1 tbsp. Everything Seasoning

Directions:

1. Preheat the oven to 400°F.
2. In a microwave-safe bowl, combine the mozzarella and labneh cheeses.
3. Microwave for 30 seconds, stir, then microwave for another 30 seconds. Stir well.
4. If not melted completely, microwave for another 10 to 20 seconds.
5. Add the almond flour, egg, baking powder, and salt to the bowl and mix well. Form into a dough using a spatula or your hands.
6. Cut the dough into 8 roughly equal pieces and form it into balls.
7. Roll each dough ball into a cylinder, then pinch the ends together to seal.
8. Place the dough rings in a nonstick donut pan or arrange them on a parchment paper–lined baking sheet. Sprinkle with the seasoning and bake for 12 to 15 min. or until golden brown.
9. Store in plastic bags in the freezer and defrost overnight in the refrigerator.
10. Reheat in the oven or toaster for a quick grab-and-go breakfast.

Nutrition: Calories 241 - Fats 19 g - Carbs 5.5 g - Fiber 2.5 g - Proteins 12 g

43. HAM AND SPINACH OMELET

Prep. Time: 25 Min.   **Cooking Time**: 2min.   **Servings**: 2

Ingredients:

- 1/4 Cup Ham, Chopped
- 1/4 Tsp. Black Pepper
- 1 Tbsp. Olive Oil
- 3 Eggs
- 2 Tbsps. Heavy Cream
- 1/2 Tsp. Cayenne Pepper
- 1 Tbsp. Butter
- 1/4 Cup Spinach, Chopped
- 1/2 Tsp. Italian Seasoning
- 1/4 Cup Cheddar Cheese
- 1/4 Tsp. Salt

Directions:

1. Take a bowl and put the eggs, salt, cayenne pepper, Italian seasoning, and black pepper in it. Whisk it well and add in cheese and cream as well. Mix well.
2. Take a pan and put olive oil and half tsp butter in it. Heat it and sauté the diced ham and spinach in it. Once they become soft, reduce the heat.
3. Add the egg mixture in it cook both sides of the omelet for a few min.
4. Take out once done and sprinkle parsley on top.

Nutrients: Calories: 362 kcal Fat: 32g Carbohydrates: 1g Protein: 16g Cholesterol: 307g

44. BREAKFAST HASH

Prep. Time: 20 Min.   **Cooking Time**: 4 Min.   **Servings**: 4

Ingredients:

- 1 Tbsp. Olive Oil
- 1 Turnip, Peeled & Diced
- 1 Tbsp. Parsley
- 1/4 Onion, Diced
- 1 Cup Brussel Sprouts, Halved
- 1/2 Tsp. Black Pepper
- 1/2 Tsp. Salt
- 3 Slices Bacon, Chopped
- 1/4 Cup Red Bell Pepper, Diced
- 1/2 Tsp. Paprika
- 1/2 Tsp. Garlic Powder

Directions:

1. Take a skillet and heat the olive oil in it over medium heat. Sauté the turnip in it along with all the spices for about 6 min.
2. Put the Brussel sprouts and onion in it and cook for another 3 min., until they become soft.
3. Add in the chopped bacon and bell pepper. Sauté it until the bacon is cooked through.
4. Once done, dish out and sprinkle chopped parsley on top.

Nutrients: Calories: 126 kcal Fat: 9g Carbohydrates: 3g Protein: 7g Fiber: 2g

45. BACON WRAPPED EGG CUPS

Prep. Time: 30 Min.   **Cooking Time**: 27 Min.   **Servings**: 12

Ingredients:

- 12 Eggs
- 2 Cups Bacon Strips
- Black Pepper, To Taste
- Cooking Spray

Directions:

1. Preheat the oven to 400 degrees F and spray on a muffin tin with cooking spray.
2. Lay the bacon strips in the muffin tin in a basket shape, covering all the sides and cut the extra bacon.
3. Put the muffin tin in the preheated oven for 5-7 min., do not overcook.
4. Take the tray out of the oven and crack one egg in every bacon basket.
5. Bake for another 10-15 min. and take out of the oven.
6. Serve the bacon egg cups with a sprinkle of black pepper on top.

Nutrients: Calories: 126 kcal Fat: 8g Carbohydrates: 0g Protein: 9g Fiber: 0g

46. GRANOLA CLUSTERS

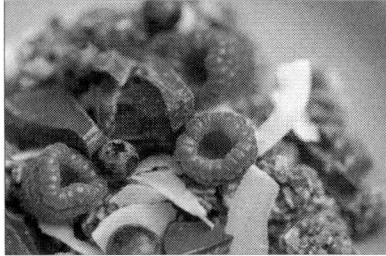

Prep. Time: 45 Min. **Cooking Time**: 30 Min. **Servings**: 8

Ingredients:
- 1/2 Cup Butter
- 1 Cup Pecan Halves
- 1/2 Cup Almonds
- 1/4 Cup Swerve Brown
- 1 Cup Coconut, Flaked
- 1/2 Cup Pumpkin Seeds
- 1/2 Tsp. Vanilla Extract
- 1/4 Cup Swerve Sweetener, Powdered
- 1/2 Tsp. Salt

Directions:
1. Preheat the oven to 300 degrees F.
2. Put the salt, pumpkin seeds, coconut, pecans, and almonds in a blender and blend for a few min. until they are crumbled.
3. Heat the butter in a saucepan with sweeteners and stir well, until the butter melts. Take off the heat and stir in the vanilla extract. Add in the nut mixture in it and mix well. Put the mixture on a parchment paper-lined a baking sheet and lay down the mixture on it. Put another parchment paper on top and with a rolling pin roll it down to a uniform thickness.
4. Put the baking sheet in the preheated oven and bake until it becomes golden, for about 20-30 min.
5. Take out of the oven once done and cool down on a wire rack.
6. Break with hands into granola clusters and store for up to a week in an airtight container.

Nutrients: Calories: 327 kcal Fat: 31.5g Carbohydrates: 6 Protein: 5.5g Fiber: 3.5g

47. DEVILED EGGS WITH BACON

Prep. Time: 15 Min. **Cooking Time**: 5 Min. **Servings**: 4

Ingredients:
- 12 Eggs
- 1/2 Tsp. Paprika Powder
- 1 Cup Bacon Slices
- 1/2 Cup Mayonnaise
- Parsley, Fresh & Chopped
- 1 Tbsp. Dijon Mustard
- Sea Salt, To Taste
- 1/2 Tsp. Olive Oil
- Black Pepper, To Taste

Directions:
1. Boil the eggs as you like them and put them under cold water to peel them easily.
2. Heat olive oil in a pan and stir fry the bacon slices in it over medium-high flame for about 5 min., until they are cooked through and become crispy. Chop the cooked bacon into small pieces. Cut the peeled eggs into halves lengthwise and take out the yolks.
3. Put the egg yolks in a bowl and add in the mayonnaise, bacon pieces, Dijon mustard, paprika powder, salt, and black pepper. Mix them well to combine.
4. Fill the egg whites hollows with a spoonful of this mixture and sprinkle chopped parsley on top.

Nutrients: Calories: 70 kcal Fat: 41g Carbohydrates: 1g Protein: 25g

48. CRUSTLESS QUICHE RECIPE

Prep. Time: 35 Min. **Cooking Time**: 25 Min. **Servings**: 6

Ingredients:
- 5 Eggs
- 1/2 Cup Cherry Tomatoes, Chopped
- 1/2 Cup Milk

- 1/2 Cup Broccoli, Chopped
- 1/2 Cup Half and Half
- 1/2 Cup Bacon, Chopped
- 2/3 Cup Mozzarella Cheese, Shredded
- 1/4 Tsp Black Pepper, Ground
- 1/2 Tsp Salt
- Cooking Spray

Directions:
1. Preheat the oven to 325 degrees F.
2. Take a baking dish (9-inches) and spray it with cooking spray.
3. Scatter the chopped bacon, broccoli, and tomatoes on it, evenly.
4. Take a bowl and crack the eggs in it. Add in the half-and-half, milk, salt, and pepper, and whisk them well to combine.
5. Pour this egg mixture over the scattered veggies and bacon in the baking dish.
6. Top it with shredded mozzarella cheese and put it in the preheated oven.
7. Bake it until the cheese is golden from the top and everything is cooked through, for about 25 min. Once done, take out and let cool for a few min., then serve.

Nutrients: Calories: 216 kcal Fat: 17g Carbohydrates: 4g Protein: 11g Fiber: 1g

49. SIMPLE FLUFFY PANCAKES

Prep Time: 5 Min.   **Cooking Time**: 15 Min.   **Servings**: 8

Ingredients:
- 1 egg
- 1¼ cups coconut milk
- 3 tbsp. butter, melted
- ½ cup coconut flour
- 3½ tsp.s baking powder
- ¼ tbsp. stevia
- 1 tsp. salt

Directions:
1. Whisk together the egg, coconut milk, and butter in a large bowl. Combine the flour, baking powder, stevia, and salt in a separate bowl. Pour the flour mixture into the egg mixture. Keep whisking until lumps are gone.
2. Warm a lightly greased baking pan over medium heat for 10 min. Make a pancake: Pour ¼ cup of the mixture in the pan and cook for 3 min. or until bubbly Flip the pancake over and cook for another 3 min. until fluffy.
3. Transfer the pancake onto a platter and allow to cool until ready to serve. Repeat with the remaining mixture.
4. You can top the pancake with different berries to add it all kinds of flavor.

Nutrients: Calories: 171 Total Fat: 14.6g Carbs: 9.5g Protein: 2.8g Cholesterol: 89mg Sodium: 346mg

50. STIR-FRIED TOMATO AND SCRAMBLED EGGS

Prep Time: 10 Min.   **Cooking Time**: 8 Min.   **Servings**: 4

Ingredients:
- 4 eggs, beaten
- 2 tomatoes, chopped
- 1 tbsp. butter
- ¼ cup onion, chopped
- 2 tbsp. feta cheese, crumbled
- Salt and ground black pepper, to taste

Directions:
1. Put the butter into a nonstick skillet and melt over medium heat, then tilt the skillet so the butter coats the bottom evenly.
2. Add the chopped onion into the skillet and stir-fry for 3 min. or until the onion is translucent, then add the beaten eggs and stir-fry for 3 min. to scramble the eggs, and then add the tomatoes, cheese, salt, and ground black pepper and stir-fry for 2 min. more until the cheese melts.
3. Transfer the scrambled eggs with tomatoes to a ceramic plate and serve.
4. To make this a complete meal, serve it with stir-fried pork chops or roast beef.

Nutrients: Calories: 116 Total Fat: 9.1g Carbs: 2g Protein: 6.8g Cholesterol: 198mg Sodium: 435mg

51. SWEET AND SOUR PANCAKES

Prep. Time: 10 Min.   **Cooking Time:** 20 Min.   **Servings:** 4
Ingredients:

- ¾ cup coconut milk
- 2 tbsp. white vinegar
- 1 egg, beaten
- 2 tbsp. butter, melted
- ¼ cup coconut flour or almond flour
- ½ tsp. baking soda
- 1 tsp. baking powder
- ¼ tsp. liquid stevia
- ½ tsp. salt

Directions:

1. Mix the milk with white vinegar in a bowl. Let it sit for 5 min. for turning 'sour', then pour the beaten egg and melted butter into the bowl. Stir to mix well.
2. In a separate bowl, mix the coconut flour, baking soda, baking powder, stevia, and salt, then pour the flour mixture into the milk mixture. Fully stir until smooth, but avoid over-mixing. Warm a lightly greased baking pan over medium heat for 10 min. To make a pancake, pour ¼ cup of the mixture in the pan and cook for 3 min. or until bubbles form on top. Flip the pancake over and cook for another 3 min. until lightly browned.
4. Transfer the pancake onto a platter and allow to cool until ready to serve. Repeat with the remaining mixture.
5. You can top the pancake with different berries to add it all kinds of flavor.

Nutrients: Calories: 216 Total Fat: 19.0g Carbs: 8.7g Protein: 4.2 Cholesterol: 170mg Sodium: 526mg

52. KETO ALMOND CREPES

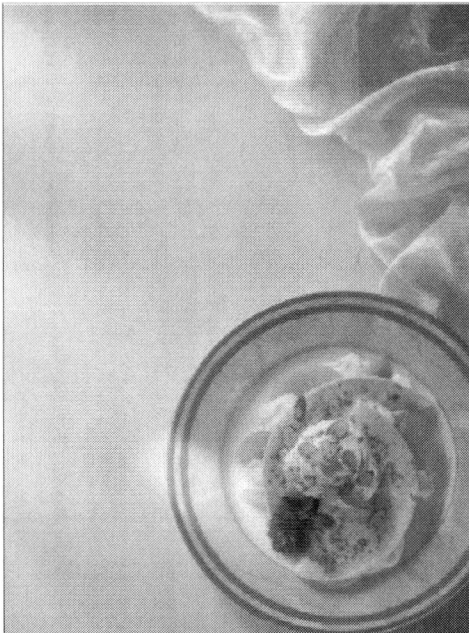

Prep. Time: 35 Min.   **Cooking Time:** 5 Min.
Servings: 8 To 10 Crepes
Ingredients:

- 4 Eggs
- 1 Tsp. Olive Oil
- 1/2 Cup Cream Cheese, Softened
- 1/4 Cup Almond Milk, Unsweetened
- 2 Tbsps. Swerve Sweetener, Granulated
- 3/4 Cup Almond Flour
- 1/8 Tsp. Salt

Directions:

1. Combine all the ingredients in a blender, except oil. Blend until a smooth consistency is attained.
2. Heat olive oil in a pan over medium-low flame and put this egg mixture in it. Swirl the pan to spread the batter evenly.
3. Cook both sides to golden brown and dish out.
4. Serve with any low carb spread of your choice.

Nutrients: Calories: 158 kcal Fat: 13g Carbohydrates: 3.04g Protein: 6.28g Fiber: 1.16g

CHAPTER 9: APPETIZER AND SNACKS

53. CARAMELIZED BUTTER WITH CREAMY EGGS

Prep Time: 10 Min.   **Cooking Time**: 15 Min.   **Servings**: 4

Ingredients:

- 1.5 pounds (680 g) green asparagus
- 2 ounces (57 g) butter, melted
- 4 eggs
- ½ cup sour cream
- 3 ounces (85 g) Parmesan cheese, grated
- Salt and cayenne pepper, to taste
- 1 tbsp. olive oil
- 3 ounces (85 g) butter
- 1½ tbsp. lemon juice

Directions:

1. Put the melted 2 ounces butter in a nonstick skillet and tilt the pan so the butter coats the bottom evenly. Separate the eggs into the skillet and stir-fry over medium heat for 3 min. or until the eggs are scrambled.
2. Transfer the scrambled eggs into a blender, then add the sour cream and cheese. Process until the mixture is creamy, then sprinkle the salt and cayenne pepper to season.
3. Clean the skillet and drizzle with olive oil, then add the asparagus, salt, and cayenne pepper and roast over medium heat for 2 or 3 min. or until soft. Flip the asparagus constantly during the cooking. Remove from the skillet and set aside.
4. Clean the skillet and put in 3 ounces butter, then sauté for 8 min. or until the butter is browned and smells nutty.
5. Add the lemon juice and cooked asparagus into the skillet and sauté with the browned butter for 2 to 3 min. until warmed through.
6. Transfer to a serving plate, and top with creamy eggs before serving.

Nutrients: Calories: 518 Total Fat: 47g Net Carbs: 6g Fiber: 4g Protein: 18 g

54. BACON-WRAPPED JALAPEÑO

Prep Time: 10 Min.   **Cooking Time**: 10 Min.   **Servings**: 6

Ingredients:

- 12 slices bacon
- 6 fresh jalapeño peppers, halved lengthwise and deseeded
- 1 (8 ounces / 227 g) package cream cheese

SPECIAL EQUIPMENT:

- 6 toothpicks

Directions:

1. On a clean working surface, scatter the cream cheese on top of the jalapeño pepper halves.
2. Wrap each pepper half with a slice of bacon and use a toothpick to secure. Repeat with the remaining pepper half and bacon slices.
3. Arrange the bacon-wrapped jalapeño on a preheated grill and grill for 8 min., flipping the bacon halfway through or until lightly browned.
4. Remove from the grill and discard the toothpick. Allow to cool before serving.

Nutrients: Calories: 391 Total Fat: 38.3g Carbs: 2.2g Protein: 9.5g Cholesterol: 79mg Sodium: 577mg

55. CHEESY SPINACH BROWNIES

Prep Time: 20 Min.   **Cooking Time**: 35 Min.   **Servings**: 24

Ingredients:

- 1 (10-ounce / 284 g) package spinach, blanched and chopped
- 1 cup almond flour
- 1 tsp. gluten-free baking powder
- 1 tsp. salt
- 2 eggs, beaten
- 1 cup unsweetened almond milk
- ½ cup butter, melted
- 1 (8 ounces / 227 g) package mozzarella cheese, shredded
- 1 onion, chopped

Directions:

1. Start by preheating the oven to 375°F (190°C).
2. Make the brownies: Combine the flour, baking powder, and salt in a bowl. Fold in the beaten eggs, almond milk, and melted butter. Then add the spinach, cheese, and onion. Stir to combine.

3. Pour the mixture into a lightly greased baking pan. Arrange the pan in the oven and bake for 30 min. or until a toothpick inserted in the center of the brownies comes out clean.
4. Remove from the oven. Allow to cool for a few min. and slice to serve.

Nutrients: Calories: 92 Total Fat: 6g Carbs: 5.6g Protein: 4.1g Cholesterol: 32mg Sodium: 216mg

56. CLOUD BREAD AND BLT

Prep Time: 25 Min.   **Cooking Time**: 20 Min.   **Servings**: 2

Ingredients:

CLOUD BREAD:
- 3 eggs
- 1 pinch salt
- ¼ tsp. cream of tartar (optional)
- ½ tbsp. ground psyllium husk powder
- 4 ounces (113 g) cream cheese
- ½ tsp. gluten-free baking powder

FILLING:
- 1 tomato, thinly sliced
- 2 ounces (57 g) lettuce, chopped
- 4 tbsp. sugar-free mayonnaise
- 5 ounces (142 g) bacon, cooked and diced

Directions:

1. Start by preheating the oven to 300°F (150°C).
2. Separate the eggs into a bowl of egg whites and another bowl of egg yolk. Sprinkle the egg whites with salt and cream of tartar, whip until puffed.
3. Then add the psyllium husk powder, cream cheese, and baking powder in the whipped egg whites. Pour the egg white mixture into the egg yolks, stir to mix well.
4. Line a baking pan with parchment paper, spoon two dollops on the mixture on the paper. Use a spatula to

form dollops of the mixture into ½-inch (1.3 cm) thick.
5. Arrange the pan in the preheated oven and bake for 25 min., flipping the cloud bread halfway through the cooking time or until golden brown. Repeat with the remaining mixture and make two cloud bread more.
6. Assemble two pieces of the cloud breads with the ingredients for the filling according to your favorite order before serving.

Nutrients: Calories: 800 Total Fat: 75g Net Carbs: 7g Fiber: 3g Protein: 22g

57. FRIED BACON AND EGGS

Prep Time: 10 Min.   **Cooking Time**: 10 Min.   **Servings**: 4

Ingredients:

- 4 ounces (113 g) bacon, in slices
- 4 eggs
- Salt and ground black pepper, to taste

Directions:

1. Cook the bacon in a nonstick skillet over medium-high heat for 3 to 4 min. When it starts to buckle and curl, loosen and flip the bacon slice so that it browns evenly and cook for another 3 to 4 min.
2. Transfer the cooked bacon into a plate lined with paper towels. Leave the fat rendered from the bacon in the pan.
3. Break the eggs into the pan and fry over medium heat until they reach your desired

doneness. Flip the eggs halfway through. You may need to work in batches to avoid overcrowding.
4. Add the bacon in the pan and cook with eggs, then sprinkle with salt and ground black pepper to taste and cook for an additional 1 min.
5. Serve them warm on a platter.
6. You can serve this dish with halved cherry tomatoes and chopped fresh parsley.

Nutrients: Calories: 272 Total Fat: 22g Net Carbs: 1g Fiber: 0g Protein: 15g

58. GUACAMOLE

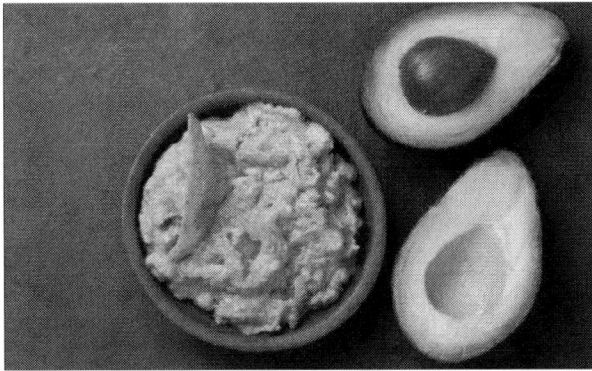

Prep Time: 10 Min.   **Cooking Time**: 0 Min.
Servings: 4

Ingredients:

- 3 avocados, peeled, pitted, and mashed
- 1 lime, juiced
- 1 tsp. salt
- 2 tbsp. (plum) tomatoes, diced
- 3 tbsp. fresh cilantro, chopped
- ½ cup onion, diced
- 1 tsp. garlic, minced
- 1 pinch ground cayenne pepper (optional)

Directions:

1. Combine the mashed avocados, lime juice, and salt in a large bowl, then fold in the tomato dices, chopped cilantro, diced onion, minced garlic, and cayenne pepper. Stir to combine well.
2. Wrap the bowl in plastic and store in the fridge for at least 1 hour before serving.

Nutrients: Calories: 262 Total Fat: 22.3g Carbs: 18g Protein: 3.8g Cholesterol: 0mg Sodium: 596mg

59. HALLOUMI CHEESE WITH SCRAMBLED EGGS

Prep Time: 10 Min.   **Cooking Time**: 15 Min.   **Servings**: 2

Ingredients:

- 3 ounces (85 g) halloumi cheese, diced
- 4 ounces (113 g) bacon, diced
- 4 eggs
- 4 tbsp. fresh parsley, chopped
- Salt and ground black pepper, to taste
- 2 scallions, chopped
- 2 ounces (57 g) olives, pitted

Directions:

1. Whisk together the eggs, parsley, salt, and ground black pepper in a medium bowl. Set aside.
2. Cook the bacon in a nonstick skillet over medium-high heat for 3 to 4 min. When it starts to buckle and curl, loosen and flip the bacon slice so that it browns evenly and cook for another 3 to 4 min.
3. Use the spatula to dice the bacon, then add the halloumi cheese and scallions, cook for 1 min. more.
4. Add the egg mixture and olives into the skillet, then turn down the heat and sauté over medium heat for 3 min. until the eggs are scrambled. Serve them on a platter immediately. To make this a complete meal, you can serve it with a bowl of cauliflower rice.

Nutrients: Calories: 657 Total Fat: 59g Net Carbs: 4g Fiber: 1g Protein: 28 g

60. JALAPEÑO PEPPERS STUFFED WITH SAUSAGE

Prep Time: 15 Min.   **Cooking Time**: 7 Min.   **Servings**: 12 Pcs

Ingredients:

- 1 pound (454 g) large fresh jalapeño peppers, halved lengthwise and deseeded
- 1 pound (454 g) ground pork sausage
- 1 cup Parmesan cheese, shredded
- 1 (8 ounces / 227 g) package cream cheese, softened
- 1 (8 ounces / 227 g) bottle Ranch dressing (optional)

Directions:

1. Start by preheating the oven to 425°F (220°C).
2. Sauté the ground pork sausage in a nonstick skillet over medium-high heat for 6 min. or

until lightly browned. Transfer to a plate lined with paper towels.

3. Combine the sautéed sausage with Parmesan cheese and cream cheese. Scoop 1 tbsp. of this mixture into each jalapeño half, then place them into a greased baking pan. You may need to work in batches to avoid overcrowding. Transfer the pan into the preheated oven.

4. Bake for 20 min. or until the jalapeño peppers are blistered and the sausage mixture are well browned, then top them with Ranch dressing, if desired, and bake for 2 min. more.

5. Remove from the oven. Allow to cool for a few min. before serving.

Nutrients: Calories: 362 Total Fat: 34.3g Carbs: 4.3g Protein: 9.2g Cholesterol: 58mg Sodium: 601mg

61. KETO BACON AND SPINACH FRITTATA

Prep Time: 10 Min.   **Cooking Time:** 35 Min.   **Servings:** 4

Ingredients:
- 8 ounces (227 g) fresh spinach, chopped
- 5 ounces (142 g) bacon
- 2 tbsp. butter
- 8 eggs, beaten
- 1 cup heavy whipping cream
- 5 ounces (142 g) mozzarella cheese, shredded
- Salt and ground black pepper, to taste

Directions:
1. Start by preheating the oven to 350°F (180°C).
2. Cook the bacon in a nonstick skillet over medium-high heat for 3 to 4 min. When it starts to buckle and curl, loosen and flip the bacon slice so that it browns evenly and cook for another 3 to 4 min.
3. Use spatula to dice the bacon, then add the butter into the skillet and melt. Tilt the skillet so the butter coat the bottom evenly.
4. Add the spinach into the skillet and sauté until wilted, then transfer them into a greased baking pan.

5. To make the frittata, combine the beaten eggs and cream in a bowl, then pour the mixture into the pan. Arrange the pan in the preheated oven. Bake the frittata for 25 min. You can check the doneness by cutting a small slit in the center, if raw eggs run into the cut, baking for another few min.
6. Sprinkle with mozzarella cheese, salt, and ground black pepper, and bake for another 2 min. until the cheese milts.
7. Remove the frittata from the oven, Allow to cool for a few min. before serving.

Nutrients: Calories: 661 Total Fat: 59g Net Carbs: 4g Fiber: 1g Protein: 27g

62. MUSHROOM AND ONION OMELET

Prep Time: 5 Min.   **Cooking Time:** 10 Min.   **Servings:** 1

Ingredients
- 4 large mushrooms, sliced
- ¼ cup yellow onion, chopped
- 3 eggs
- Salt and ground black pepper, to taste
- 1 ounce (28 g) butter, melted
- 1 ounce (28 g) Cheddar cheese, shredded

Directions:
1. Whisk the eggs in a large bowl, and sprinkle with salt and ground black pepper. Stir until frothy. Set aside.
2. Drizzle the melted butter in a nonstick skillet. Tilt the pan so the butter covers the bottom evenly. sauté the mushrooms and yellow onion in the skillet over medium-high heat for 3 min. until the mushrooms are tender and onion is translucent.

3. To make the omelet, pour the egg mixture over the skillet and cook for 1 to 2 min. until the omelet starts to firm, then flip the omelet, sprinkle with Cheddar cheese, and cook for another 1 min.
4. Gently fold the omelet in half with a spatula and transfer to a plate to cool before serving.
5. To make it a complete meal, you can serve the

omelet with seasoned bacon rolls and avocado wedges.

Nutrients: Calories: 517 Total Fat: 44g Net Carbs: 5g Fiber: 1g Protein: 26 g

63. PARMESAN ASPARAGUS

Prep Time: 10 Min.   **Cooking Time:** 15 Min.   **Servings:** 4

Ingredients

- 1 ounce (28 g) shaved Parmesan cheese
- 1 pound (454 g) thin asparagus spears
- 1 tbsp. extra virgin olive oil
- Freshly ground black pepper, to taste

Directions:

1. Start by preheating the oven to 450°F (220°C).
2. Coat a baking pan with olive oil, then place the asparagus spears into the pan. Sprinkle with Parmesan cheese and ground black pepper.
3. Arrange the pan in the preheated oven and cook for 12 min. until the asparagus spears are crisp and tender, and the cheese melts.
4. Remove them from the oven. Allow to cool for a few min. before serving.
5. To make this a complete meal, serve it with balsamic vinegar or other sugar-free sauces on top, which can increase the flavor of this recipe.

Nutrients: Calories: 93 Total Fat: 5.6g Carbs: 7g Protein: 5.3g Cholesterol: 6mg Sodium: 114 mg

64. SHRIMP SKEWERS

Prep Time: 70 Min.   **Cooking Time:** 0 Min.   **Servings:** 6

Ingredients

- 2 pounds (907 g) fresh shrimp, peeled and deveined
- 2 tbsp. red wine vinegar
- ¼ cup unsweetened tomato sauce
- 3 cloves garlic, minced
- ⅓ cup olive oil
- 2 tbsp. fresh basil, chopped
- ½ tsp. salt
- ¼ tsp. cayenne pepper

SPECIAL EQUIPMENT: 6 skewers, soaked in water for at least 30 min. to avoid them from burning

Directions:

- Combine the red wine vinegar, tomato sauce, garlic, and olive oil in a large bow. Put the peeled and deveined shrimps in the bowl, and sprinkle with basil, salt, and cayenne pepper. Toss to coat well.
- Wrap the bowl in plastic and refrigerate to marinate for at least 1 hour.
- Discard the marinade. Thread the shrimps through the skewers, then arrange the shrimp skewers onto the preheated grill.
- Grill for 6 min. Flip halfway through the cooking time or until opaque. Serve warm.
- To make this a complete meal, you can serve the shrimp skewers with a veggie salad.

Nutrients: Calories: 273 Total Fat: 14.7g Carbs: 2.8g Protein: 31g Cholesterol: 230mg Sodium: 472 mg

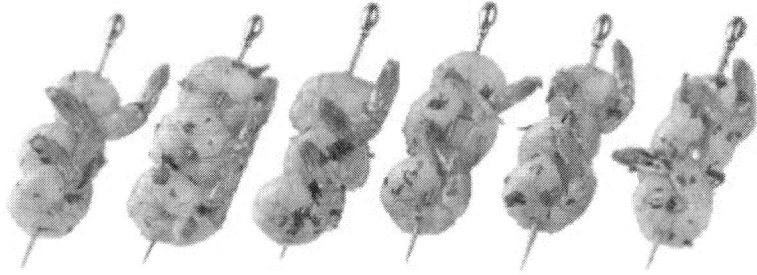

CHAPTER 10: LUNCH RECIPES

65. MEDITERRANEAN TUNA SALAD WITH OLIVES

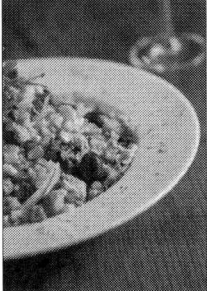

Prep. Time: 10 Min.   **Cooking Time:** 7 Min.   **Servings:** 1

Ingredients

- 1 & 1/2 tsp Lemon juice, or to taste
- 1 Can Tuna, packed in water (5 oz. Drained)
- 1 Tbsp Paleo Mayo
- 1 Tbsp Sun-Dried Tomatoes Packed in Olive Oil, drained and diced
- 1 tsp Lemon zest
- 1 tsp Pine nuts
- 1/2 tsp Dried parsley
- 1/4 tsp Dried Basil
- 1/4 tsp dried oregano
- 2 Tbsp Roasted red peppers, sliced
- 4 Cherry Tomatoes, diced
- 4 Kalamata olives, sliced
- Salt, to taste

Directions:

1. Take oven to 350 °F.
2. On a small baking sheet, cook around 5-7 min. until the pine nuts turn to a light brown color. Don't burn them.
3. Put all ingredients in the mug and stir. Use salt as seasoning and taste with lemon juice.
4. Chop and mix the pine nuts into the tuna.
5. Serve in wraps of lettuce or on toast.

Nutrients: Calories: 351 kcal Fat: 20g Carbohydrates: 13.2g Protein: 35.2g Fiber: 2.9g

66. KETO GREEN BEAN CASSEROLE

Prep. Time: 50 Min.   **Cooking Time:** 40 Min.   **Servings:** 6

Ingredients

- 1 1/4 tsp. Sea salt
- 1 cup Onion, diced
- 2 cups Green beans, trimmed
- 1/3 cup 2% milk (or 1/2 cup almond milk)
- 1/4 Cup Full fat cream cheese (dairy-free works too)
- 1/4 tsp. Pepper
- 2 Cups Mushrooms, sliced
- 2/3 cup Half and half cream (or 1/2 cup full-fat coconut milk)
- 6 Slices Bacon

Directions:

1. Heat the oven to 350°F. Take a frying pan over medium heat. Cook until the bacon turns to golden brown color and crispy on sides.
2. Then remove excess fat after transferring it to a paper towel. Reserve only 1 Tbsp. of fat.
3. Add onions & mushrooms in a medium to high heated pan. Cook until golden brown by stirring sporadically for about 3 min.
4. Boil all ingredients except beans.
5. Boil for 4 min. until the mixture thickens by stirring continuously. Cook by stirring continuously on reduced heat, and cook until mixture is very thick, for 7-8 min. Boil salted water in a large pot. Cook green beans until they become fork tender. It should take 7-8 min. Dry them by draining excess water and patting them with a paper towel.
6. Then, add cooked beans into the sauce and stir to coat beans with sauce.
7. Put into a pan of size 8x8 inch and cook for 15-20 min.
8. While you are cooking beans, make crumbs of bacon in a food processor. Use casserole to sprinkle and bake for 5 min.

Nutrients: Calories: 159 kcal Fat: 11g Carbohydrates: 10.3g Protein: 6.2g Fiber: 3.3g

67. KETO CHICKEN TACO SOUP

Prep. Time: 25 min.   **Cooking Time**: 15 min.   **Servings**: 4

Ingredients

- shredded cheddar cheese optional
- fresh sliced jalapeño optional
- 8 oz full-fat cream cheese room temperature
- 4 tbsp fresh chopped cilantro optional
- 3 tbsp Low Carb Taco Seasoning
- 3 cups chicken broth
- 1 lime, cut into wedges optional
- 2 cups chicken breast tenders
- 1 cup of salsa

Directions:

1. Take an instant pot and put the chicken broth, taco seasoning, and chicken in it.
2. Make sure that the release valve is sealed. Choose a cycle time of about 15 min. in manual mode. The cycle will start automatically. Once the cycle is completed, let it for 10 min. Then release the valve.
3. Take chicken out of the pot and use a fork to shred it. Choose sauté setting on the instant pot. Whisk the cream with chicken broth mixture. Simmer the shredded chicken in the pot for about 3-4 min.
4. If desired, top with cilantro, cheddar cheese shredded, lime wedge, and jalapeño.

Nutrients: Calories: 215 kcal Fat: 10.62g Carbohydrates: 10.75g Protein: 16.2g Fiber: 2.1g

68. CRUNCHY ASIAN CABBAGE SALAD

Prep. Time: 50 min.   **Cooking time**: 0-min.   **Servings**: 4

Ingredients

For Salad Dressing
- 1 tsp Bragg's Amino Acids
- 1 tsp Dijon Mustard
- 2 tbsp Rice Wine Vinegar
- 1/4 cup Coconut Oil Liquid

Cabbage
- 1/4 tsp Freshly Cracked Pepper
- 3 tbsp Rice Wine Vinegar
- 1/2 head Green Cabbage Cored and finely shredded
- 1/2 tsp Kosher Salt
- 1/2 cup Coconut Oil Liquid

Cucumbers
- 1/4 cup Cilantro Chopped with no stems
- 1/2 Hothouse Cucumber Seeded
- 1 tbsp Sesame Seeds (Optional)
- 1/4 Fresh Red Chili Pepper (Optional) Sliced thin

- 1/4 tsp Kosher Salt
- 1 tbsp Olive Oil

Red peppers (Asian)
- 2 tsp Sesame Oil
- 1 Red Pepper cored, seeded, and sliced very thin
- 1/2 tsp Ginger Fresh, from a jar or 1/4 tsp dried ginger
- 1/4 cup Scallion Greens Sliced or
- 1/4 tsp Ground Cumin
- 2 tbsp finely diced shallots.

Remaining Ingredients
- 1 Avocado Peeled, sliced and seeded
- 1 cup Snow Pea Pods

Optional Quick Pickled Onions
- 2 tbsp Red Wine Vinegar
- 1/4 cup Red Onion Finely diced

Directions

Asian cabbage
1. Take a large bowl and shred the cabbage in it. Mix well after adding the remaining ingredients.
2. Don't let it sit at the bottom.

Asian cucumbers

1. Take a medium bowl and slice cucumbers in it.
2. Put rest of the ingredients and rest it for 30 min.

Asian red peppers

1. Take a medium bowl and slice red peppers in it.
2. Put rest of the ingredients and rest it for 30 min.

Quick Pickled Onions

1. Take a medium bowl and diced onions in it.
2. Take red wine vinegar and cover the onions with it.
3. Rest it for 20 min.

Salad Dressing

1. Take a bowl and add all the ingredients.

2. Set it aside at room temperature after mixing.

Cabbage Salad

1. After marinating all the ingredients of the salad, put the cabbage in a bowl.
2. Top it with equal portions of marinated red peppers, marinated cucumber, and sliced avocado. (In the case of snow peas, put peas into the salad.)
3. Whereas, in the case of pickled onions, top them with a pinch of cilantro.
4. And to garnish, use sesame seeds.

Nutrients: Calories: 519 kcal Fat: 52g Carbohydrates: 10g Protein: 2.2g Fiber: 2.9g

69. KETO DUTCH BABY WITH CHOCOLATE AND MACADAMIA

Prep. Time: 20 min.   **Cooking Time**: 0-min.   **Servings**: 4

Ingredients

- 4 large eggs
- 2 tbsp coconut flour
- 2 tbsp butter
- 1/8 tsp salt
- 1/4 cup monk fruit sweetener
- 1/4 cup heavy whipping cream
- 1/4 cup almond flour
- 1/2 cup sugar-free whipped cream optional
- 1/2 cup strawberries optional
- 1 tsp vanilla extract
- 1 tbsp sugar-free chocolate syrup

Directions

1. Preheat the oven to 400°F.
2. Put butter (2 tbsps.) in a preheated oven.
3. In a large bowl, whisk together 1/4 cup Sweetener (Monk fruit), 2 tbsp coconut flour, 1/8 tsp salt, and 1/4 cup almond flour.
4. In a second bowl, add 1 tsp vanilla extract, 4 large eggs, and 1/4 cup heavy whipped cream.
5. Stir until well combined.
6. Combine mixtures of egg and almond flour.
7. Remove skillet from the oven and pour batter (Dutch Baby) in skillet.
8. Bake skillet in the oven for 15 min. to brown the Dutch Baby top.
9. Take 1 tbsp. ChocZero syrup and drizzle the pancake.
10. Take 1 tbsp. nuts (macadamia) and sprinkle the pancake. Serve with fresh strawberries and sugar-free whipped cream.

Nutrients: Calories: 272 kcal Fat: 23.62g Carbohydrates: 8.74g Protein: 8.52g Fiber: 5.7g

70. EASY KETO SMOKED SALMON LUNCH BOWL

Prep. Time: 15 Min.   **Cooking Time**: 0 Min.   **Servings**: 2

Ingredients:

- 12 ounces smoked salmon
- 4 tbsp. mayonnaise
- 2 ounces spinach
- 1 tbsp. olive oil
- 1 medium lime
- Salt and pepper

Directions:

1. Arrange the mayonnaise, salmon, spinach on a plate.
2. Sprinkle olive oil over the spinach.
3. Serve with lime wedges and put salt plus pepper.

Nutrition: Calories 457 - Fats 34.8 g - Carbs 1.9 g - Proteins 32.3 g

71. EASY ONE-PAN GROUND BEEF AND GREEN BEANS

Prep. Time: 15 Min.   **Cooking Time:** 15 Min.   **Servings:** 2

Ingredients:

- 10 ounces ground beef
- 9 ounces green beans
- Salt and pepper
- 2 tbsp. sour cream
- 3½ ounces butter

Directions:

1. Warm-up the butter to a pan over high heat.
2. Put the ground beef plus the pepper and salt. Cook.
3. Reduce heat to medium.
4. Add the remaining butter and the green beans then cook within five min.
5. Put pepper and salt, then transfer.
6. Serve with a dollop of sour cream.

Nutrition: Calories 787 - Fats 71.7 g - Carbs 6.65 g - Proteins 27.5 g

72. EASY SPINACH AND BACON SALAD

Prep. Time: 15 Min.   **Cooking Time:** 15 Min.   **Servings:** 4

Ingredients:

- 8 ounces spinach
- 4 large, hard-boiled eggs
- 6 ounces bacon
- 2 medium red onions
- 2 cups of mayonnaise
- Salt and pepper

Directions:

1. Cook the bacon, then chop into pieces, set aside.
2. Slice the hard-boiled eggs, and then rinse the spinach.
3. Combine the lettuce, mayonnaise, and bacon fat into a large cup, put pepper and salt.
4. Add the red onion, sliced eggs, and bacon into the salad, then toss. Serve.

Nutrition: Calories 509 - Fats 45.9 g - Carbs 2.5 g - Proteins 19.7 g

73. EASY KETO ITALIAN PLATE

Prep. Time: 15 Min.   **Cooking Time:** 0 Min.   **Servings:** 2

Ingredients:

- 7 ounces mozzarella cheese
- 7 ounces prosciutto
- 2 tomatoes
- 4 tbsp. olive oil
- 10 whole green olives
- Salt and pepper

Directions:

1. Arrange the tomato, olives, mozzarella, and prosciutto on a plate.
2. Season the tomato and cheese with pepper and salt. Serve with olive oil.

Nutrition: Calories 780 - Fats 60.7 g - Carbs 5.9 g - Proteins 50.8 g

74. FRESH BROCCOLI AND DILL KETO SALAD

Prep. Time: 15 Min.   **Cooking Time:** 7 Min.   **Servings:** 3

Ingredients:

- 16 ounces broccoli
- 1/2 cup mayonnaise
- 3/4 cup chopped dill
- Salt and pepper

Directions:

1. Boil salted water in a saucepan.
2. Put the chopped broccoli in the pot and boil for 3-5 min.
3. Drain and set aside.
4. Once cooled, mix the rest of the fixing.
5. Put pepper and salt, then serve.

Nutrition: Calories 303 - Fats 28.1 g - Carbs 6.2 g - Proteins 4 g

75. PARMESAN ROASTED RANCH CAULIFLOWER WITH AVOCADO

Prep. Time: 35 Mins　　　**Cooking Time:** 12 Min.　　　**Servings:** 4

Ingredients

- 2 Tbsp. Olive oil
- 2 cups Cauliflower, cut into large florets
- 1 large avocado, cubed
- 2 Tbsp. Finely grated Parmesan cheese
- 2 Tbsp. Ranch mix (recipe below)
- Pinch of sea salt

Ranch Seasoning:

- 3/4 tsp Salt
- 1 Tbsp Dried Parsley
- 1 tsp Garlic powder
- 1/3 tsp Pepper
- 1 tsp Onion powder
- 1 tsp Dried Dill

Directions:

1. Preheat the oven to 400°F.
2. Take a bowl, mix the oil and cauliflower in it.
3. Add 2 Tbsp. of mixed ranch mix to cauliflower. Coat by tossing. Spread a single layer of cauliflower on a baking sheet. Leave space between the flowers.
4. First, cook for 15 min. and then cook again for 12 min. after stirring until the color changes to Golden Brown.
5. Toss with avocado, cheese, and some salt in a bowl.

Nutrients: Calories: 179 kcal Fat: 14.5g Carbohydrates: 11g Protein: 5g Fiber: 6.5g

76. SPINACH SALAD WITH WARM BACON DRESSING

Prep. Time: 30 mins　　　**Cooking Time:** 6 min.　　　**Servings:** 4

Ingredients

- 2 oz Mushrooms, sliced very thinly (about 4 large)
- oz Baby Spinach
- 4 large, boiled eggs, chopped
- 8 oz Bacon, diced

Warm Bacon Dressing

- 1/4 cup bacon grease
- 2 tbsp Red wine vinegar
- 1 tbsp Low carb brown sugar
- 2 tbsp Shallot, finely chopped
- Salt and pepper to taste
- 1/2 tsp Dried tarragon
- 1 tbsp Whole Grain Mustard

Customize

- Mandarin oranges, apple, walnuts, strawberries, shrimp, blue cheese

Directions:

1. Put diced bacon in a pan on medium heat.
2. Cook for 5-6 min. by stirring sporadically.
3. Pour bacon oil into a small bowl after removing it from the pan.
4. Chop or slice the eggs, mushrooms, and shallot. Heat mushrooms in a pan over medium heat to lightly cook them.
5. Take shallots and sauté them.
6. Turn the heat to medium-low and add the Sukrin Gold, bacon oil, tarragon, vinegar, and whole grain mustard. Combine all of these by stirring continuously. Add pepper and salt to taste.
7. Toss the hot dressing with the spinach and divide between 4 serving bowls. Taste to adjust seasoning. Top with bacon, eggs, and mushrooms.

Nutrients: Calories: 445 kcal | Fat: 32g | Carbohydrates: 5.14g | Protein: 28g | Fiber: 1.8g

77. CHICKEN COBB SALAD WITH COBB SALAD DRESSING

Prep. Time: 20 mins　　　**Cooking Time:** 0-min.　　　**Servings:** 2

Ingredients

- 4 oz cooked chicken breast, diced (about 1 medium breast)
- 180 grams romaine lettuce, chopped (2 hearts of romaine)
- 2 large boiled eggs, quartered, sliced, or chopped

- 6 tbsp Cobb Salad Dressing (or blue cheese dressing)
- 2 oz cheddar cheese, cubed
- 4 slices cooked bacon, crumbled
- 2-3 green onions, sliced
- 1/2 Hass avocado, cubed or sliced

Directions:
1. Take lettuce and toss it with cobb salad dressing.
2. Divide it into 2 bowls.
3. Serve

Nutrients: Calories: 632 kcal Fat: 54g Carbohydrates: 9.5g Protein: 29g Fiber: 5g

78. BROCCOLI CHEDDAR QUICHE WITH BACON

Prep. Time: 50 mins   **Cooking Time:** 40 min.   **Servings:** 6

Ingredients
- 1/4 cup almond milk (or water)
- 6 large eggs
- 1/4 cup raw onions, finely chopped (1 ounce)
- 1 1/4 cup heavy cream
- 2 cups shredded cheddar cheese (8 ounces)
- 1/4 tsp salt
- 6 oz bite-sized broccoli florets (steamed until crisp-tender)
- 1/4 tsp white pepper
- 4 slices cooked bacon, crumbled

Directions:
1. Preheat oven to 350°F.
2. Spray a baking spry on a 10" plate.
3. Cook the bacon and crumble it.
4. Now, steam broccoli. And dice onions.
5. Layer the ingredients on a quiche plate: 1/3 each of the broccoli, onion, 1/4 of the cheese, and bacon.
6. Add the almond milk, heavy cream, salt, eggs, and pepper to a medium bowl and use a hand mixer to beat it.
7. Then, take custard and pour over the quiche ingredients. Bake it for 40 min. to brown the top. Serve.

Nutrients: Calories: 457 kcal Fat: 40g Carbohydrates: 3.8g Protein: 20g Fiber: 0.5g

79. AVOCADO CHICKEN SALAD

Prep. Time: 15 mins   **Cooking Time:** 0 min.   **Servings:** 3

Ingredients
- 1 medium Hass Avocado, mashed
- 2 cups poached chicken diced (10 oz)
- 1/3 cup celery, finely diced (1 large rib)
- 2 tbsp cilantro, finely chopped
- salt and pepper to taste
- 2 tbsp red onion or scallion, minced
- 1 tbsp fresh lemon juice (or lime juice)
- 2 tbsp avocado oil (or your favorite)

Directions:
1. Prepare the onion, celery, and cilantro in a bowl. Take diced chicken and vegetables in the bowl. Cut avocado in half. Then scoop the flesh from the avocado.
2. Use a fork to mash it and turn it to smoot and creamy texture.
3. Take oil and lemon juice and stir the ingredients.
4. Add all ingredients together in a bowl and mix by stirring. Serve with lettuce.

Nutrients: Calories: 267 kcal Fat: 20g Carbohydrates: 4g Protein: 19g Fiber: 1g

80. KETO SMOKED SALMON FILLED AVOCADOS

Prep. Time: 15 Min.   **Cooking Time:** 0 Min.   **Servings:** 1

Ingredients:
- 1 avocado
- 3 ounces smoked salmon
- 4 tbsp. sour cream

- 1 tbsp. lemon juice
- Salt and pepper

Directions:
1. Cut the avocado into two.
2. Place the sour cream in the hollow parts of the avocado with smoked salmon.
3. Put pepper and salt, squeeze lemon juice over the top.
4. Serve.

Nutrition: Calories 517 - Fats 42.6 g - Carbs 6.7 g - Proteins 20.6 g

81. LOW-CARB BROCCOLI LEMON PARMESAN SOUP

Prep. Time: 15 Min   **Cooking Time:** 15 Min.   **Servings:** 4

Ingredients:
- 3 cups of water
- 1 cup unsweetened almond milk
- 32 ounces broccoli florets
- 1 cup heavy whipping cream
- 3/4 cup Parmesan cheese
- Salt and pepper
- 2 tbsp. lemon juice

Directions:
1. Cook broccoli plus water over medium-high heat. Take out 1 cup of the cooking liquid, and remove the rest.
2. Blend half the broccoli, reserved cooking oil, unsweetened almond milk, heavy cream, and salt plus pepper in a blender.
3. Put the blended items to the remaining broccoli, and stir with Parmesan cheese and lemon juice.
4. Cook until heated through. Serve with Parmesan cheese on the top.

Nutrition: Calories 371 - Fats 28.3 g - Carbs 11.6 g - Proteins 14.6 g

82. PROSCIUTTO AND MOZZARELLA BOMB

Prep. Time: 15 Min.   **Cooking Time:** 10 Min.   **Servings:** 4

Ingredients:
- 4 ounces sliced prosciutto
- 8 ounces mozzarella ball
- Olive oil

Directions:
1. Layer half of the prosciutto vertically.
2. Lay the remaining slices horizontally across the first set of slices. Place mozzarella ball, upside down, onto the crisscrossed prosciutto slices.
3. Wrap the mozzarella ball with the prosciutto slices.
4. Warm-up the olive oil in a skillet, crisp the prosciutto, then serve.

Nutrition: Calories 253 - Fats 19.3 g - Carbs 1.1 g - Proteins 18 g

83. TUNA AVOCADO SALAD

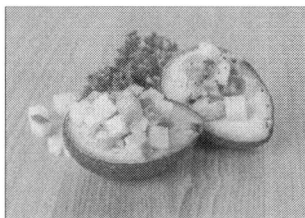

Prep. Time: 15 Min.   **Cooking Time:** 0 Min.   **Servings:** 2

Ingredients:
- 1 can tuna flake
- 1 medium avocado
- 1 medium English cucumber
- ¼ cup cilantro
- 1 tbsp. lemon juice
- 1 tbsp. olive oil
- Salt and pepper

Directions:
1. Put the first 4 ingredients into a salad bowl.
2. Sprinkle with lemon and olive oil.
3. Serve.

Nutrition: Calories 303 - Fats 22.6 g - Carbs 5.2 g - Proteins 16.7 g

84. MUSHROOMS & GOAT CHEESE SALAD

Prep. Time: 15 Min   **Cooking Time**: 10 Min.   **Servings**: 1

Ingredients:

- 1 tbsp. butter
- 2 ounces cremini mushrooms
- Salt and pepper
- 4 ounces spring mix
- 1-ounce cooked bacon
- 1-ounce goat cheese
- 1 tbsp. olive oil
- 1 tbsp. balsamic vinegar

Directions:

1. Sautee the mushrooms, put pepper and salt.
2. Place the salad greens in a bowl. Top with goat cheese and crumbled bacon.
3. Mix these in the salad once the mushrooms are done.
4. Whisk the olive oil in a small bowl and balsamic vinegar.
5. Put the salad on top and serve.

Nutrition: Calories 243 - Fats 21 g - Carbs 8 g - Fiber 1 g - Proteins 11.6 g

85. KETO BACON SUSHI

Prep. Time: 15 Min.   **Cooking Time**: 13 Min.   **Servings**: 4

Ingredients:

- 6 slices bacon
- 1 avocado
- 2 Persian cucumbers
- 2 medium carrots
- 4 oz. cream cheese

Directions:

1. Warm-up oven to 400F. Line a baking sheet.
2. Place bacon halves in an even layer and bake, 11 to 13 min.
3. Meanwhile, slice cucumbers, avocado, and carrots into parts roughly the width of the bacon.
4. Spread an even layer of cream cheese in the cooled-down bacon.
5. Divide vegetables evenly and place them on one end. Roll up vegetables tightly.
6. Garnish and serve.

Nutrition: Calories 343 - Fats 30 g - Carbs 11.6 g - Proteins 28 g

86. LOW CARB CHICKEN SOUP

Prep. Time: 30 mins   **Cooking Time**: 5 min.   **Servings**: 6

Ingredients

- 6 cups bone broth
- 2 cups cooked chicken, diced

Vegetable Base

- 1 cup celery, sliced
- 4 tbsp butter, avocado oil, or olive oil
- 1/2 cup onion, diced
- 1 large garlic clove, sliced
- 8 ounces celery root, cubed
- 1 whole bay leaf
- 1/3 cup carrot
- 2 tsp chicken base
- 1 tsp lemon zest
- 2 tsp lemon juice mixed with water
- salt and pepper to taste
- 1 tbsp garlic herb seasoning blend
- 1/4 cup dry white wine

Directions:

1. Take diced chicken. Take vegetables. Peel and cut them.
2. Add butter, lemon zest, bay leaf, and vegetables in a quart pot on medium heat.
3. Stir continuously to coat everything.
4. Add chicken base, wine, and garlic herb blend after reducing the heat to medium.
5. Cook vegetables for about 3-4 min. until they turn brown.
6. Boil the chicken broth, then simmer the vegetables over reduced heat until they become tender. Add the chicken broth and bring it to just under a boil. Add pepper and salt to taste.

Nutrients: Calories: 274 kcal Fat: 15 Carbohydrates: 8g Protein: 26g Fiber: 2g

87. SWEET AND SOUR GERMAN GREEN BEANS WITH BACON AND ONIONS

Prep. Time: 18 mins   **Cooking Time:** 5 Min.   **Servings:** 4

Ingredients

- 4 slices bacon, diced
- 2 cups green beans
- 2 tbsp apple cider vinegar
- 1/4 cup onion, finely chopped
- 1 tbsp Low carb brown sugar
- 2 tbsp water
- 1 tsp wholegrain mustard
- 1/4 tsp salt

Directions:

1. Take trimmed beans, chopped onions, and diced bacon.
2. Turn beans tender by cooking.
3. Cook bacon in a pan over medium heat for 4 min.
4. Sauté the onions.
5. Add the Sukrin Gold, water, onions, and cider vinegar to the bacon.
6. Take a pan and put grain mustard in it.
7. At last, take green beans and coat by stirring at heat thoroughly.
8. Use pepper and salt to taste.

Nutrients: Calories: 166 kcal Fat: 11g Carbohydrates: 8g Protein: 9g Fiber: 4g

88. THAI CHICKEN SATAY WITH PEANUT SAUCE

Prep. Time: 35 mins   **Cooking time:** 0 mins   **Servings:** 4

Ingredients

- 2 cups chicken tenders

Chicken Satay Marinade
- 1 tbsp Hot Madras Curry Powder
- 1/3 cup full fat coconut milk from a can
- 1/4 cup chopped fresh cilantro (optional)
- 1/2 tsp ground coriander

- 2 tbsp Red Boat Fish Sauce (optional)
- 2 tbsp Low carb brown sugar

Peanut Sauce
- 1/3 cup full fat coconut milk from a can
- 1 tsp soy sauce
- 1/4 cup smooth peanut/almond butter

- 1-2 tsp chile-garlic sauce
- 1 tbsp Low carb brown sugar
- 1/2 tsp Thai Red Curry Paste

Extras
- soaked bamboo skewers
- lime wedges
- chopped fresh cilantro

Directions:

1. take warm water and soak the skewers in it.
2. Cut the chicken in half and place it in zip-lock bags. Take the satay marinade in a bowl and put a chicken in it to coat all sides of the chicken. Marinate overnight or for 30 min.
3. Warm peanut butter in a small bowl.
4. Whisk in the chile-garlic sauce, Sukrin Gold, Thai curry paste, and soy sauce.
5. Then, add coconut milk slowly. Season it to taste. Refrigerate it.
6. Thread the chicken tenders onto the bamboo skewers.
7. Cook the chicken on the grill, either indoor or outdoor.
8. Garnish it with fresh cilantro (chopped).
9. Serve with the peanut sauce and a lime wedge.

Nutrients: Calories: 279 kcal Fat: 15g Carbohydrates: 4g Protein: 30g Fiber: 1g

89. FAJITA HASSELBACK CHICKEN

Prep. Time: 5 mins   **Cooking Time:** 20 mins   **Servings:** 4

Ingredients

- ½ red bell pepper, diced
- 4 chicken breasts
- ½ yellow bell pepper, diced

- ½ onion, diced
- 2 Tbsps. fajita spice mix
- ½ cup cheddar cheese (50 g), grated

> ☞ 3 Tbsps. salsa

> ☞ ½ green pepper, diced

Directions:

1. Take the oven to 350°F.
2. Cut and slice the chicken but not deep enough to keep the bottom intact.
3. Take fajita mix, and mix the cooked onions and pepper on medium heat.
4. Take salsa and stir in the mixture. Use cheese to sprinkle over it. Melt the cheese and mix all ingredients. Fill chicken slices with 1 tbsp of mixture.
5. Bake the chicken in the oven for 20 min., and juice run through it.

Nutrients: Calories: 368 Fat: 11g Carbohydrates: 9g Protein: 53g Fiber: 1g

90. CHICKEN SPINACH BLUEBERRY SALAD WITH PARMESAN CHEESE

Prep. Time: 20 mins   **Cooking Time:** 0 mins   **Servings:** 2

Ingredients

Chicken Spinach Blueberry Salad

> ☞ 6 cups baby spinach (170 g)

> ☞ 8 ounces chicken tenders or chicken breast

> ☞ 4 cups fresh blueberries

> ☞ Two slices of red onion (paper-thin)

> ☞ 2 cups shaved Parmesan cheese

> ☞ 1 cup sliced almonds (toasted or raw)

Balsamic Dressing

> ☞ 1 tbsp red wine vinegar

> ☞ 1/4 cup extra light olive oil

> ☞ 1 tbsp balsamic vinegar

> ☞ 2 tsp minced red onion

> ☞ 1/2 tsp dijon mustard

> ☞ 1 tbsp water

> ☞ 1 pinch each salt and pepper

> ☞ 1/8 tsp dried thyme

> ☞ 1/2 tsp low carb sugar

Method

1. Grill the chicken thoroughly. And cut it into small pieces. Take almonds, and minced the onions, and make the dressing (balsamic).
2. Brown the almonds slightly in a frying pan. Cool it after removing it from the pan.
3. Add all ingredients of the dressing and blend them well with a stick blender.
4. Take spinach and arrange it evenly on two plates.

Nutrients: Calories: 519 kcal Fat: 38g Carbohydrates: 10g Protein: 35g Fiber: 4g

91. COLE SLAW KETO WRAP

Prep. Time: 15 Min.   **Cooking Time:** 0 Min.   **Servings:** 2

Ingredients:

> ☞ 3 c Red Cabbage

> ☞ 5 c Green Onions

> ☞ 75 c Mayo

> ☞ 2 tsp Apple Cider Vinegar

> ☞ 25 tsp Salt

> ☞ 16 pcs Collard Green

> ☞ 1-pound Ground Meat, cooked

> ☞ .33 c Alfalfa Sprouts

> ☞ Toothpicks

Directions:

1. Mix slaw items with a spoon in a large-sized bowl.
2. Place a collard green on a plate and scoop a tbsp. of coleslaw on the edge of the leaf.
3. Top it with a scoop of meat and sprouts.
4. Roll and tuck the sides.
5. Insert the toothpicks.
6. Serve.

Nutrition: Calories 409 - Fats 42 g - Carbs 4 g - Fiber 2 g - Proteins 2 g

92. KETO CHICKEN CLUB LETTUCE WRAP

Prep. Time: 15 Min.   **Cooking Time:** 15 Min.   **Servings:** 1

Ingredients:

> ☞ 1 head iceberg lettuce

> ☞ 1 tbsp. mayonnaise

> ☞ 6 slices of organic chicken

> ☞ Bacon

🏳 Tomato

Directions:
1. Layer 6-8 large leaves of lettuce in the center of the parchment paper, around 9-10 inches.
2. Spread the mayo in the center and lay with chicken, bacon, and tomato.
3. Roll the wrap halfway through, then roll tuck in the ends of the wrap.
4. Cut it in half.
5. Serve.

Nutrition: Calories 837 - Fats 78 g - Carbs 4 g - Fiber 2 g Proteins 28 g

93. KETO BROCCOLI SALAD

Prep. Time: 10 Min.   **Cooking Time:** 0 Min.   **Servings:** 4-6

Ingredients:

For salad:

🏳 2 broccoli

🏳 2 red cabbage

🏳 .5 c sliced almonds

🏳 1 green onion

🏳 .5 craisins

For the orange almond dressing:

🏳 33 c orange juice

🏳 25 c almond butter

🏳 2 tbsp. coconut aminos

🏳 1 shallot

🏳 Salt

Directions:
1. Pulse the salt, shallot, amino, nut butter, and orange juice using a blender.
2. Combine other fixing in a bowl.
3. Toss it with dressing and serve.

Nutritional: Calories 202 - Fats 9.4 g - Carbs 1.3 g - Fiber 0.3 g - Proteins 2.2 g

94. KETO SHEET PAN CHICKEN AND RAINBOW VEGGIES

Prep. Time: 15 Min   **Cooking Time:** 25 Min.   **Servings:** 4

Ingredients:

🏳 Nonstick spray

🏳 1-pound Chicken Breasts

🏳 1 tbsp. Sesame Oil

🏳 2 tbsp. Soy Sauce

🏳 2 tbsp. Honey

🏳 2 Red Pepper

🏳 2 Yellow Pepper

🏳 3 Carrots

🏳 ½ Broccoli

🏳 2 Red Onions

🏳 2 tbsp. EVOO

🏳 Pepper & salt

🏳 .25 c Parsley

Directions:
1. Grease the baking sheet, warm-up the oven to a temperature of 400°F.
2. Put the chicken in the middle of the sheet.
3. Separately, combine the oil and the soy sauce.
4. Brush over the chicken.
5. Separate veggies across the plate.
6. Sprinkle with oil and then toss.
7. Put pepper & salt.
8. Set tray into the oven and cook within 25 min.
9. Garnish using parsley.
10. Serve.

Nutrition: Calories 437 - Fats 30 g - Carbs 9 g - Fiber 0.5 g - Proteins 30 g

95. SHRIMP LETTUCE WRAPS WITH BUFFALO SAUCE

Prep. Time: 15 Min.   **Cooking Time:** 20 Min.   **Servings:** 4

Ingredients:

🏳 1 egg, beaten

🏳 3 Tbsp. butter

🏳 16 oz. shrimp, peeled, deveined, with tails removed

🏳 ¾ cup almond flour

🏳 ¼ cup hot sauce (like Frank's)

🏳 1 tsp extra-virgin olive oil

🏳 Kosher salt

- Black pepper
- Garlic
- 1 head romaine lettuce, leaves parted, for serving
- ½ red onion, chopped
- celery, finely sliced
- ½ blue cheese, cut into pieces

Directions:

1. To make the Buffalo sauce, melt the butter in a saucepan, add the garlic and cook this mixture for 1 min. Pour hot sauce into the saucepan and whisk to combine. Set aside.
2. In one bowl, crack one egg, add salt and pepper and mix. In another bowl, put the almond flour, add salt and pepper and also combine. Dip each shrimp into the egg mixture first and then into the almond one.
3. Take a large frying pan. Heat the oil and cook your shrimp for about 2 min. per side.
4. Add Buffalo sauce.
5. Serve in lettuce leaves. Top your shrimp with red onion, blue cheese, and celery.

Nutrition: Calories 606 - Fats 54 g - Carbs 8 g - Proteins 33 g

96. POKE BOWL WITH SALMON AND VEGGIES

Prep. Time: 20 Min.　　**Cooking Time:** 0 Min.　　**Servings:** 2

Ingredients:

- 8 oz. raw salmon, skinless and deboned
- 1 Tbsp. sesame oil
- 1 tsp tamari sauce
- 1 pinch salt
- 1 cup white cabbage, shredded
- 1 cup red cabbage, shredded
- ¼ cup cucumber, sliced
- 1 radish, sliced
- ½ avocado, diced
- ¼ cup cilantro
- 1 tsp white sesame seeds
- 1 tsp black sesame seeds

Directions:

1. To make the marinade, mix the sesame oil, tamari sauce and salt. Set aside.
2. Cut your salmon into cubes and put it into a bowl.
3. Pour the marinade over it.
4. Place the cucumber, red and white cabbage, radish, avocado and cilantro into a bowl.
5. Add the marinated salmon.
6. Top the salmon with white and black sesame seeds.

Nutrition: Calories 446 - Fats 34 g - Carbs 11 g - Proteins 26 g

97. KETO TUNA MELT

Prep. Time: 15 mins　　**Cooking Time:** 5 mins　　**Servings:** 4

Ingredients

- 3 Tbsps. Mayonnaise
- 1.5 cups Canned Tuna
- ¼ cup Sliced celery
- 1 Tbsp. Finely diced red onion
- 4 slices Cheddar Cheese
- 2 Tbsps. Dill pickle relish
- ¼ Tsp. Salt
- 4 Tomato slices from a large tomato

Directions:

1. Take a bowl. Add and stir mayonnaise, tuna, celery, red onion, and dill relish.
2. Sprinkle some salt on the tomato slices placed on a baking sheet. Then, on each slice, add 1/4 of the tuna mixture.
3. Take slices of cheese to top each tomato slice.
4. Cook until cheese melts. It should take about 3-5 min.
5. Serve

Nutrients: Calories: 227 kcal Fat: 14g Carbohydrates: 3g Protein: 21g Fiber: 1g

98. CHEESY BAKED ZUCCHINI CASSEROLE

Prep. Time: 45 mins　　**Cooking Time:** 30 mins　　**Servings:** 6

Ingredients

- 2 Tbsps. Butter

- 4.5 cups (approximately) zucchini, large, sliced 1/4 inch thick
- 1/2 cups Onion, diced
- 1 Tsp. Salt
- 1/2 cups Parmesan Cheese, grated and divided
- ½ cup Heavy Cream
- 2 cloves garlic, minced
- 1/2 cups Gruyere Cheese, grated and divided

Directions:

1. Heat the oven to 450°F.
2. Prepare and pace the salted zucchini slices on a paper towel.
3. Let sit each side for 15 min. each.
4. Put zucchini slices on a dish.
5. Take a skillet and heat the butter to melt it.
6. Then add onion and garlic to cook them for 3 min. and 2 min., respectively.
7. Add the heavy cream while stirring in a pan.
8. Add Gruyere cheese and Parmesan cheese and melt the cheese while stirring.
9. Add the sauce (cheese) to the zucchini.
10. Bake zucchini with parmesan and Gruyere for 5 min. by covering the casserole dish with a foil. Remove it when tender.
11. Serve.

Nutrients: Calories: 275 kcal Fat: 21g Carbohydrates: 7g Protein: 13g Fiber: 1g

99. MEXICAN KETO MEATBALLS

Prep. Time: 50 mins   **Cooking Time**: 30mins   **Servings**: 15 meatballs

Ingredients

- 2 Tbsps. Chili Powder
- 2 Tsps. Salt
- 2 Tbsps. Cumin
- 2 cups Ground Beef
- 1/4 cup Jalapeños, finely diced
- 1 Egg
- 85 g Cheddar Cheese, shredded

Directions:

1. Take oven to 400°F.
2. Take a large bowl and mix every ingredient in it.
3. Bake balls of 2-inch size after rolling meat in balls like shape.
4. For 25-30 min., bake them on a sheet (baking).

Nutrients (2 meatballs): Calories: 220 kcal Fat: 18g Carbohydrates: 2 Protein: 14g Fiber: 2g

100. MEAT LOVERS' STUFFED PEPPERS

Prep. Time: 1 hr 10 mins   **Cooking time**: 40mins   **Servings**: 6

Ingredients

- 225 g Mozzarella cheese
- 50 g Pepperoni small pieces
- 3 Bell peppers, any color
- ¾ cup Pasta sauce
- Cooked 175 g Italian sausage

Directions

1. Heat oven to 400°F. Cut pepper and place them on the dish after removing seeds in them.
2. On the bottom side of each pepper, put 1 tbsp. Sauce.
3. Use pepperoni pieces and 30 g of Italian sausage as a topping.
4. Put some mozzarella.
5. Put sauce, pepperoni, and mozzarella again as the topping. Make sure to fill pepper with enough mozzarella.
6. Bake peppers in the oven for 40 min. until cheese is melted.

Nutrients: Calories: 284 kcal Fat: 22g Carbohydrates: 6g Protein: 16g Fiber: 2g

101. SHORT RIBS

Prep. Time: 2 hrs 30 mins   **Cooking Time**:   **Servings**: 4

Ingredients

- Kosher salt
- 4 cups Short Ribs
- 1 Tbsp. Olive Oil
- Pepper
- 2 sprigs Rosemary
- 2 Bay Leaves
- 1 Onion, cut into quarters
- 4 sprigs thyme
- 3 large Carrots, cut into quarters
- 2-4 cups Beef Broth
- ½ cup Red Wine

Directions

1. Put pepper and salt on all sides of the ribs.
2. Add olive oil 1 tbsp. in the pot on sauté setting. Brown sides of ribs, it takes 2 min. for each side. Set aside beef ribs.
3. Cook onions and carrots in the pot for 5 min. Cook with red wine.
4. Put herbs wrapped in cheesecloth with onions and carrots in a pressure cooker.
5. Now, Put beef ribs in the pot.
6. Take out the broth in another pot.
7. For 1.5 hours, cook everything in a pressure cooker on high pressure.
8. When done, release the pressure.
9. Strain vegetables and beef in a bowl and put away herbs and vegetables.
10. Serve.

Nutrients: Calories: 363 kcal Fat: 21g Carbohydrates: 4g Protein: 33g Fiber: 1g

102. THAI CUCUMBER NOODLE SALAD

Prep. time: 10 min. **Cooking time**: 1-min. **Servings**: 3

Ingredients:

- 1 cucumber, cut into noodles
- salt, to taste
- 3 pinches scallions, chopped
- 3 pinches raisins
- 3 tsp sesame seeds
- ¼ cup unsalted almond butter
- 1 tsp red curry paste
- ¼cup canned coconut milk
- 1½ Tbsp. apple cider vinegar
- ⅛ tsp coarse salt
- 1 Tbsp. coconut water

Directions:

1. With a Julienne peeler, make noodles from the cucumber.
2. To make the Thai peanut sauce, combine and mix thoroughly the unsalted almond butter, red curry paste, canned coconut milk, apple cider vinegar, coconut water, and add coarse salt.
3. Place your cucumber noodles over a spacious flat plate, pour ½ Tbsp.
4. Thai peanut sauce over the noodles.
5. Top the cucumber noodles with chopped scallions, raisins, and sesame seeds.

Nutrition: Calories 132 - Fats 10 g - Carbs 3 g - Proteins 3 g

103. BACON CHEESEBURGER

Prep. Time: 15 Min. **Cooking Time**: 8 Min. **Servings**: 4

Ingredients:

- 7 oz. bacon
- 1½ pounds ground beef
- ½ tsp salt
- ¼ tsp pepper
- 4 oz. cheese, shredded
- 1 head iceberg or romaine lettuce, leaves parted and washed
- 1 tomato, sliced
- ¼ pickled cucumber, finely sliced

Directions:

1. Cook bacon and set aside.
2. In a separate bowl, combine ground beef, salt, and pepper.
3. Divide mixture into 4 sections, create balls and press each one slightly to form a patty.
4. Put your patties into a frying pan and cook for about 4 min. on each side. Top each cooked patty with a slice of cheese, several pieces of bacon, and pickled cucumber. Add a bit of tomato. Wrap each burger in a big lettuce leaf.

Nutrition: Calories 684 - Fats 51 g - Carbs 5 g - Proteins 48 g

104. MUSHROOM & CAULIFLOWER RISOTTO

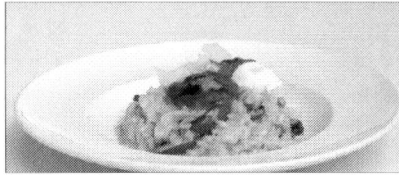

Prep Time: 5 min   **Cooking Time**: 10 min   **Servings**: 4

Ingredients:

- 1 grated head of cauliflower
- 1 cup vegetable stock
- 9 oz. chopped mushrooms
- 2 tbsp. butter
- 1 cup coconut cream.

Directions:

1. Pour the stock in a saucepan. Boil and set aside.
2. Prepare a skillet with butter and sauté the mushrooms until golden.
3. Grate and stir in the cauliflower and stock.
4. Simmer and add the cream, cooking until the cauliflower is al dente.
5. Serve.

Nutrition: Calories: 186 Carbs: 4 g Protein: 1 g Fats: 17 g.

105. PITA PIZZA

Prep Time: 15 min   **Cooking Time**: 10 min   **Servings**: 2

Ingredients:

- ½ cup marinara sauce
- 1 low-carb pita
- 2 oz. cheddar cheese
- 14 slices pepperoni
- 1 oz. roasted red peppers.

Directions:

1. Program the oven temperature setting to 450°F.
2. Slice the pita in half and place onto a foil-lined baking tray.
3. Rub with a bit of oil and toast for one to two min.
4. Pour the sauce over the bread.
5. Sprinkle using the cheese and other toppings.
6. Bake until the cheese melts (5 min.).
7. Cool thoroughly.

Nutrition: Calories: 250 Carbs: 4 g Protein: 13 g Fats: 19 g.

106. ITALIAN STYLE HALIBUT PACKETS

Prep Time: 10 min   **Cooking Time**: 20 min   **Servings**: 4

Ingredients:

- 2 cups cauliflower florets
- 1 cup roasted red pepper strips
- ½ cup sliced sun-dried tomatoes
- 4 (4-ounce) halibut fillets
- ¼ cup chopped fresh basil
- 1 lemon juice
- ¼ cup good-quality olive oil
- Sea salt, for seasoning
- Freshly ground black pepper, for seasoning.

Directions:

1. Preheat the oven. Set the oven temperature to 400°F. Make the packets.
2. Divide the cauliflower, red pepper strips, and sun-dried tomato between the four pieces of foil, placing the vegetables in the middle of each piece.
3. Top each pile with one halibut fillet and top each fillet with equal amounts of the basil, lemon juice, and olive oil.
4. Fold and crimp the foil to form sealed packets of fish and vegetables and place them on the baking sheet. Bake. Bake the packets for about 20 min., until the fish flakes with a fork.
5. Be careful of the steam when you open the packet!
6. Serve. Transfer the vegetables and halibut to four plates, season with salt and pepper, and serve immediately.

Nutrition: Calories: 313 Fat: 14.1 g Carbs: 3.2 g Fiber: 10.4 g Protein: 15.4 g.

107. TACO CASSEROLE

Prep Time: 10 min   **Cooking Time**: 20 min   **Servings**: 8

Ingredients:

- 1½ to 2 lb. ground turkey or beef
- 8 oz. shredded cheddar cheese
- 16 oz. cottage cheese.
- 2 tbsp. taco seasoning
- 1 cup salsa

Directions:

1. Heat the oven to reach 400 °F.
2. Combine the taco seasoning and ground meat in a casserole dish.
3. Bake it for 20 min.
4. Combine the salsa and both kinds of cheese. Set aside for now.
5. Carefully transfer the casserole dish from the oven.
6. Drain away the cooking juices from the meat.
7. Break the meat into small pieces and mash with a masher or fork.
8. Sprinkle with cheese.
9. Bake in the oven for 15 to 20 more min. until the top is brown.

Nutrition: Calories: 367 kcal Carbs: 6 g Protein: 45 g Fats: 18 g.

108. BEEF WELLINGTON

Prep Time: 20 min   **Cooking Time**: 40 min   **Servings**: 4

Ingredients:

- 2 (4-ounce) grass-fed beef tenderloin steaks, halved
- Salt and ground black pepper, as required
- 1 tbsp. butter
- 1 cup mozzarella cheese, shredded
- ½ cup almond flour
- 4 tbsp. liver pate.

Directions:

1. Preheat your oven to 400°F. Grease a baking sheet. Season the steaks with pepper and salt.
2. Sear the beef steaks for about 2–3 min. per side. In a microwave-safe bowl, add the mozzarella cheese and microwave for about 1 min. Remove from the microwave and stir in the almond flour until a dough forms.
3. Place the dough between 2 parchment paper pieces and, with a rolling pin, roll to flatten it.
4. Remove the upper parchment paper piece.
5. Divide the rolled dough into four pieces.
6. Place one tbsp. of pate onto each dough piece and top with one steak piece.
7. Cover each steak piece with dough completely.
8. Arrange the covered steak pieces onto the prepared baking sheet in a single layer.
9. Baking time: 20-30 min.
10. Serve warm.

Nutrition: Calories: 412 Fat: 15.6g Carbs: 4.9 g Fiber: 9.1g Protein: 18.5g.

109. KETO CROQUE MONSIEUR

Prep Time: 5 min   **Cooking Time**: 7 min   **Servings**: 2

Ingredients:

- 2 eggs
- ¾ oz. of grated cheese
- ¾ oz. of ham 1 large slice
- 3 tbsp. of cream
- 3 tbsp. of mascarpone
- 1 oz. of butter
- Pepper and salt
- Basil leaves, optional, to garnish.

Directions:

1. Carefully crack eggs in a neat bowl, add some salt and pepper. Add the cream, mascarpone, grated cheese, and stir together.
2. Melt the butter over medium heat. The butter must not turn brown.

3. Once the butter has melted, set the heat to low.
4. Add half of the omelette mixture to the frying pan and then immediately place the slice of ham on it.
5. Now pour the rest of the omelette mixture over the ham and then immediately put a lid on it.
6. Allow it to fry for 2-3 min. over low heat until the top is slightly firmer.
7. Slide the omelette onto the lid to turn the omelette.
8. Then put the omelette back in the frying pan to fry for another 1-2 min. on the other side (still on low heat), then put the lid back on the pan. Don't let the omelette cook for too long!
9. It does not matter if it is still liquid.
10. Garnish with a few basil leaves if necessary.

Nutrition: Calories: 479 Protein: 16 g Fats: 45 g Carbs: 4 g.

110. KETO WRAPS WITH CREAM CHEESE AND SALMON

Prep Time: 5 min   **Cooking Time**: 10 min   **Servings**: 2

Ingredients:

- 3 oz. of cream cheese
- 1 tbsp. of dill or other fresh herbs
- 1 oz. of smoked salmon
- 1 egg
- ½ oz. of butter
- Pinch of cayenne pepper
- Pepper and salt.

Directions:

1. Beat the egg well in a bowl. With 1 egg, you can make two thin wraps in a small frying pan.
2. Melt the butter over medium heat in a small frying pan.
3. Once the butter has melted, add half of the beaten egg to the pan.
4. Move the pan back and forth so that the entire bottom is covered with a very thin layer of egg. Turn down the heat!
5. Carefully loosen the egg on the edges with a silicone spatula and turn the wafer-thin omelets as soon as the egg is no longer dripping (about 45 seconds to 1 min.).
6. You can do this by sliding it onto a lid or plate and then sliding it back into the pan.
7. Let the other side be cooked for about 30 seconds and then remove from the pan.
8. The omelets must be nice and light yellow.
9. Repeat for the rest of the beaten egg.
10. Once the omelets are ready, let them cool on a cutting board or plate and make the filling.
11. Cut the dill into small pieces and put in a bowl
12. Add the cream cheese, the salmon cut into small pieces, and mix together. Add a tiny bit of cayenne pepper and mix well. Taste immediately and then season with salt and pepper.
13. Spread a layer on the wrap and roll it up. Cut the wrap in half and keep in the fridge until you are ready to eat it.

Nutrition: Calories: 237 Carbs: 14.7 g Protein: 15 g Fat: 5 g.

111. SESAME PORK WITH GREEN BEANS

Prep Time: 5 min   **Cooking Time**: 10 min   **Servings**: 2

Ingredients:

- 2 boneless pork chops
- Pink Himalayan salt
- Freshly ground black pepper
- 2 tbsp. toasted sesame oil, divided
- 2 tbsp. soy sauce
- 1 tsp. Sriracha sauce
- 1 cup fresh green beans.

Directions:

1. On a cutting board, pat the pork chops dry with a paper towel. Slice the chops into strips and season with pink Himalayan salt and pepper.
2. In a large skillet over medium heat, heat one tbsp. of sesame oil. Add the pork strips and cook them for 7 min., stirring occasionally.
3. In a small bowl, mix the remaining one tbsp. of sesame oil, the soy sauce, and the Sriracha sauce. Pour into the skillet with the pork.
4. Add the green beans to the skillet, reduce the heat to medium-low, and simmer for 3 to 5 min.
5. Divide the pork, green beans, and sauce between two wide, shallow bowls and serve.

Nutrition: Calories: 387 Fat: 15.1 g Carbs: 4.1 g Fiber: 10 g Protein: 18.1 g

112. PAN-SEARED COD WITH TOMATO HOLLANDAISE

Prep Time: 10 min **Cooking Time**: 10 min **Servings**: 4

Ingredients:

- Pan-Seared Cod
- 1 pound (4-fillets) wild Alaskan Cod
- 1 tbsp. salted butter
- 1 tbsp. olive oil
- Tomato Hollandaise
- 3 large egg yolks
- 3 tbsp. warm water
- 8 oz. salted butter, melted
- ¼ tsp. salt
- ¼ tsp. black pepper
- 2 tbsp. tomato paste
- 2 tbsp. fresh lemon juice.

Directions:
1. Season both sides of the code fillet without salt, the salt will be added in the last.
2. Heat a skillet over medium heat and coat with olive oil and butter.
3. When the butter heats up, place the cod fillet in the skillet and sear on both sides for 2-3 min. Baste the fish fillet with the oil and butter mixture.
4. You will know that the cod cooked when it easily flakes when poked with a fork.
5. Melt the butter in the microwave.
6. In a double boil, beat egg yolks with warm water until thick and creamy and start forming soft peaks. Remove the double boil from the heat, gradually adding the melted butter and stirring.
7. Season.
8. Mix in the tomato paste. Stir to combine. Pour in the water and lemon juice to lighten the sauce texture.

Nutrition: Calories: 356 Fat: 16.1 g Carbs: 3.1 g Fiber: 12.3 g Protein: 18.4 g.

113. CREAMY SCALLOPS

Prep Time: 10 min **Cooking Time**: 10 min **Servings**: 4

Ingredients:

- 1 lb. scallops, rinse and pat dry
- 1 tsp. fresh parsley, chopped
- ⅛ tsp. cayenne pepper
- 2 tbsp. white wine
- ¼ cup water
- 3 tbsp. heavy cream
- 1 tsp. garlic, minced
- 1 tbsp. butter, melted
- 1 tbsp. olive oil
- Pepper
- Salt.

Direction:
1. Season scallops with pepper and salt.
2. Heat butter and oil in a pan over medium heat.
3. Add scallops and sear until browned from both sides. Transfer scallops on a plate. Add garlic in the same pan and sauté for 30 seconds.
4. Add water, heavy cream, wine, cayenne pepper, and salt. Stir well and cook until sauce thickens.
5. Return scallops to pan and stir well.
6. Garnish with parsley and serve.

Nutrition: Calories: 202 kcal Fat: 11.4 g Cholesterol: 60 mg Carbs: 3.5 g Sugar: 0.1 g Protein: 19.4 g.

114.   PERFECT PAN-SEARED SCALLOPS

Prep Time: 10 min   **Cooking Time**: 4 min   **Servings**: 4

Ingredients:

- 1 lb. scallops, rinse and pat dry
- 1 tbsp. olive oil
- 2 tbsp. butter
- Pepper
- Salt.

Direction:

1. Season scallops with pepper and salt.
2. Heat butter and oil in a pan over medium heat.
3. Add scallops and sear for 2 min. then turn to the other side and cook for 2 min. more.
4. Serve and enjoy.

Nutrition: Calories: 181 Fat: 10.1 g Cholesterol: 53 mg Carbs: 2.7 g Sugar: 0 g Protein: 19.1 g.

115.   EASY BAKED SHRIMP SCAMPI

Prep Time: 10 min   **Cooking Time**: 10 min   **Servings**: 4

Ingredients:

- 2 lb. shrimp, peeled
- ¾ cup olive oil
- 2 tsp. dried oregano
- 1 tbsp. garlic, minced
- ½ cup fresh lemon juice
- ¼ cup butter, sliced
- Pepper
- Salt.

Directions:

1. Preheat the oven to 350°F.
2. Add shrimp in a baking dish.
3. In a bowl, whisk together lemon juice, oregano, garlic, oil, pepper, salt, and pour over shrimp.
4. Add butter on top of shrimp.
5. Bake in preheated oven for 10 min. or until shrimp is cooked.
6. Serve and enjoy.

Nutrition: Calories: 708 Fat: 53.5 g Cholesterol: 508 mg Carbs: 5.3 g Sugar: 0.7 g Protein: 52.2 g.

116.   DELICIOUS BLACKENED SHRIMP

Prep Time: 10 min   **Cooking Time**: 5 min   **Servings**: 4

Ingredients:

- 1½ lbs. shrimp, peeled
- 1 tbsp. garlic, minced
- 1 tbsp. olive oil
- 1 tsp. garlic powder
- 1 tsp. dried oregano
- 1 tsp. cumin
- 1 tbsp. paprika
- 1 tbsp. chili powder
- Pepper
- Salt.

Direction:

1. In a mixing bowl, mix together garlic powder, oregano, cumin, paprika, chili powder, pepper, and salt.
2. Add shrimp and mix until well coated. Set aside for 30 min.
3. Heat oil in a pan over medium-high heat.
4. Add shrimp and cook for 2 min. Turn shrimp and cook for 2 min. more.
5. Add garlic and cook for 30 seconds.
6. Serve and enjoy.

Nutrition: Calories 252 kcal Fat: 7.1 g Cholesterol: 358 mg Carbs: 6.3 g Sugar: 0.5 g Protein: 39.6 g.

117.   LAMB CHOPS AND HERB BUTTER

Prep Time: 15 min   **Cooking Time**: 4 min   **Servings**: 4

Ingredients:

- 8 lamb chops
- 1 tbsp. olive oil
- 1 tbsp. butter
- 1 tbsp. pepper
- 1 tbsp. salt.
- For the herb butter:
- 5 ounces butter
- 1 clove garlic
- ½ tbsp. garlic powder
- 4 tbsp. parsley
- 1 tsp. lemon juice
- ⅓ tsp. salt.

Directions:

1. Season the lamb chops with pepper and salt.
2. Warm-up olive oil and butter in an iron skillet. Add the lamb chops. Fry within four minutes.
3. Mix all the listed items for the herb butter in a bowl. Cool.
4. Serve with herb butter.

Nutrition: Calories: 722.3 kcal Protein: 42.3 g Carbs: 0.4 g Fat: 61.5 g Fiber: 0.4 g.

118. PORK CHOPS IN BLUE CHEESE SAUCE

Prep Time: 5 min   **Cooking Time**: 10 min   **Servings**: 2

Ingredients:

- 2 boneless pork chops
- Pink Himalayan salt
- Freshly ground black pepper
- 2 tbsp. butter
- ⅓ cup blue cheese crumbles
- ⅓ cup heavy (whipping) cream
- ⅓ cup sour cream.

Directions:

1. Dry the pork chops and season with pink Himalayan salt and pepper.
2. In a medium skillet over medium heat, melt the butter. When the butter melts and is very hot, add the pork chops and sear on each side for 3 minutes.
3. The pork chops must be transferred to a plate and let rest for 3 to 5 minutes. In a preheated pan, melt the blue cheese crumbles, frequently stirring so they don't burn.
4. Add the cream and the sour cream to the pan with the blue cheese. Let simmer for a few minutes, stirring occasionally.
5. For an extra kick of flavor in the sauce, pour the pork-chop pan juice into the cheese mixture and stir. Let simmer while the pork chops are resting.
6. Put the pork chops on two plates, pour the blue cheese sauce over the top of each, and serve.

Nutrition: Calories: 434 kcalFat: 14.1 g Carbs: 3.1 g Fiber: 11.3 g Protein: 17.5 g.

119. BUTTERED COD

Prep Time: 5 min   **Cooking Time**: 5 min   **Servings**: 4

Ingredients:

- 1½ lb. cod fillets, sliced
- tbsp. butter, sliced
- ¼ tsp. garlic powder
- ¾ tsp. ground paprika
- Salt and pepper to taste
- Lemon slices
- Chopped parsley.

Directions:

1. Mix the garlic powder, paprika, salt, and pepper in a bowl.
2. Season cod pieces with seasoning mixture.
3. Add 2 tablespoons butter in a pan over medium heat.
4. Let half of the butter melt.
5. Add the cod and cook for 2 minutes per side.
6. Top with the remaining slices of butter.
7. Cook for 3 to 4 minutes.
8. Garnish with parsley and lemon slices before serving.

Nutrition: Calories: 295 kcal Total Fat: 19 g Saturated Fat: 11 g Cholesterol: 128 mg Sodium: 236 mg Carbs: 1.5 g Fiber: 0.7 g Sugars: 0.3 g Protein: 30.7 g.

120. SALMON WITH RED CURRY SAUCE

Prep Time: 10 min   **Cooking Time**: 22 min   **Servings**: 4

Ingredients:

- salmon fillets
- 2 tbsp. olive oil
- Salt and pepper to taste
- 1½ tbsp. red curry paste
- 1 tbsp. fresh ginger, chopped
- 14 oz. coconut cream
- 1½ tbsp. fish sauce.

Directions:

1. Preheat your oven to 350ºF. Cover baking sheet with foil. Brush both sides of salmon fillets with olive oil and season with salt and pepper. Place the salmon fillets on the baking sheet. Bake salmon in the oven for 20 minutes.
2. In a pan over medium heat, mix the curry paste, ginger, coconut cream, and fish sauce.
3. Sprinkle with salt and pepper.
4. Simmer for 2 minutes.
5. Pour the sauce over the salmon before serving.

Nutrition: Calories: 553 kcal Total Fat: 43.4 g Saturated Fat: 24.1 g Cholesterol: 78 mg Sodium: 908 mg Carbs: 7.9 g Fiber: 2.4 g Sugars: 3.6 g Protein: 37.3 g.

121.   SALMON TERIYAKI

Prep Time: 15 min   **Cooking Time**: 25 min   **Servings**: 6

Ingredients:

- 3 tbsp. sesame oil
- 2 tsp. fish sauce
- 3 tbsp. coconut amino
- 2 tsp. ginger, grated
- cloves garlic, crushed
- 2 tbsp. xylitol
- 1 tbsp. green lime juice
- 2 tsp. green lime zest
- Cayenne pepper to taste
- salmon fillets
- 1 tsp. arrowroot starch
- ¼ cup of water
- Sesame seeds.

Directions:

1. Preheat your oven to 400ºF.
2. Combine the sesame oil, fish sauce, coconut amino, ginger, garlic, xylitol, green lime juice, zest, and cayenne pepper in a mixing bowl.
3. Create 6 packets using foil. Add half of the marinade in the packets.Add the salmon inside.
4. Place in the baking sheet and cook for about 20 to 25 minutes.
5. Add the remaining sauce in a pan over medium heat.
6. Dissolve the arrowroot in water and add to the sauce.
7. Simmer until the sauce has thickened.
8. Place the salmon on a serving platter and pour the sauce on top.
9. Sprinkle sesame seeds on top before serving.

Nutrition: Calories: 312 kcal Total Fat: 17.9 g Saturated Fat: 2.6 g Cholesterol: 78 mg Sodium: 242 mg Carbs: 3.5 g Fiber: 0.1 g Sugars: 0.1 g Protein: 34.8 g.

122.   GROUND BEEF STROGANOFF

Prep Time: 10 min   **Cooking Time**: 15 min   **Servings**: 4

Ingredients:

- 2 tbsp. butter
- 1 clove minced garlic
- 1 pound 80% lean ground beef
- Salt and pepper, to taste
- oz. sliced mushrooms
- 2 tbsp. water
- 1 cup sour cream
- 1 tbsp. fresh lemon juice
- 1 tbsp. fresh chopped parsley

Directions:

1. The butter must be added to a pan. When the butter has melted and stops foaming, add the minced garlic to the skillet.
2. Cook the garlic until fragrant, then mix in the ground beef—season with salt and pepper.

3. Cook the ground beef until no longer pink; break up the grounds with a wooden spoon.
4. Add the water and mushrooms to the pan and cook over medium heat.
5. Cook until the liquid has reduced halfway, and the mushrooms are tender. Set the cooked mushrooms aside.

6. Reduce the heat, then whisk the sour cream and paprika into the skillet.
7. Stir in the cooked beef and mushrooms into the pan and combine. Stir in the lemon juice and parsley.

Nutrition: Calories: 380 Fat: 15.1g Fiber: 3.6g Carbs:12.3 g Protein: 15.4g.

CHAPTER 11: DINNER RECIPES

123.   104. CRAB MELT

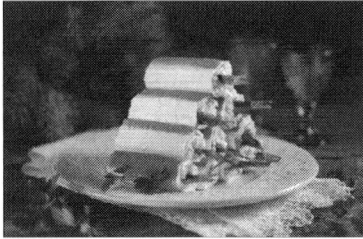

Prep. Time: 5 Min.   **Cooking Time:** 20 Min.   **Servings:** 4

Ingredients:

- 2 zucchini
- A single tbsp. of olive oil
- 3 ounces of stalks from celery
- 3/4 cup of mayo
- 12 ounces of crab meat
- A single red bell pepper
- 7 ounces of cheese (use shredded cheddar)
- A single tbsp. of Dijon mustard

Directions:

1. Preheat your oven to 450°F.
2. Slice your zucchini lengthwise.
3. Go for about a half-inch thick.
4. Add salt.
5. Let it sit for 15 min.
6. Pat it dries with a paper towel.
7. Place your slices on a baking sheet.
8. The baking sheet needs to be lined with parchment paper. Brush olive oil on each side.
9. Finely chop the vegetables.
10. Mix with the other ingredients.
11. Apply the mix to zucchini.
12. Bake for 20 min.
13. Your top will be golden brown.

Nutrition: Calories 542 - Fats 45 g - Carbs 7 g - Fiber 3 g - Proteins 20 g

124.   SPINACH FRITTATA

Prep. Time: 10 Min.   **Cooking Time:** 35 Min.   **Servings:** 4

Ingredients:

- 5 ounces of diced bacon
- 2 tbsp. of butter
- 8 ounces of spinach that's fresh
- 8 eggs
- A single cup of heavy whipping cream
- 5 ounce of shredded cheese

Directions:

1. Preheat your oven to 350°F and grease a 9 by 9 baking dish.
2. Fry your bacon on a heat medium until it is crispy.
3. Add your spinach and stir until it has wilted.
4. Remove pan from heat.
5. Place it to the side.
6. Whisk cream and eggs together and pour into the baking dish.
7. Add the spinach and bacon and pour the cheese on top. Put in the middle of the oven.
8. Bake a half hour.
9. It should be set in the middle.
10. The color on top should be golden brown.

Nutrition: Calories 661 - Fats 59 g - Carbs 4 g - Fiber 1 g - Proteins 27 g

125.   HALLOUMI TIME

Prep. Time: 5 Min.   **Cooking Time:** 15 Min.   **Servings:** 2

Ingredients:

- 3 ounces of halloumi cheese that have been diced
- 2 chopped scallions
- 4 ounces of diced bacon
- 2 tbsp. of olive oil
- 4 tbsp. of chopped fresh parsley
- 4 eggs
- Half a cup of pitted olives

Directions:

1. In a frying pan on medium-high heat, heat the oil. Fry the scallions, cheese, and bacon until they are nicely browned.
2. Get a bowl and whisk your eggs and parsley together.
3. Pour the egg mix into the pan over the bacon.
4. Lower heat.
5. Add olives.
6. Stir for 2 min.

Nutrition: Calories 663 - Fats 59 g - Carbs 4 g - Proteins 28 g

126. POBLANO PEPPERS

Prep. Time: 5 Min.   **Cooking Time:** 15 Min.   **Servings:** 2

Ingredients:

- A pound of grated cauliflower
- 3 ounces of butter
- 4 eggs
- 3 ounces of poblano peppers
- A single tbsp. of olive oil
- Half a cup of mayo

Directions:

1. Put your mayo in a bowl to the side.
2. Grate the cauliflower, including the stem.
3. Fry the cauliflower for 5 min. in the butter.
4. Brush the oil on the peppers.
5. Fry them until you see the skin bubble a little.
6. Fry your eggs any way you like.
7. Servings with mayo.

Nutrition: Calories 898 - Fats 87 g - Carbs 9 g - Proteins 17 g

127. HASH BROWNS

Prep. Time: 20 Min.   **Cooking Time:** 10 Min.   **Servings:** 4

Ingredients:

- 3 eggs
- A pound of cauliflower
- Half a grated yellow onion
- 4 ounces of butter

Directions:

1. Rinse the cauliflower.
2. Trim it.
3. Grate it using a food processor.
4. Add it to a bowl.
5. Add everything and mix.
6. Set aside 10 min.
7. Melt the right amount of butter on medium heat.
8. You need a larger skillet.
9. Place the mix in the pan and flatten.
10. Fry for 5 min. on each side.
11. Don't burn it.

Nutrition: Calories 282 - Fats 26 g - Carbs 5 g - Proteins 7 g

128. SALAD WITH BUTTER

Prep. Time: 5 Min.   **Cooking Time:** 10 Min.   **Servings:** 2

Ingredients:

- 10 ounces of goat cheese
- A quarter cup of pumpkin seeds
- 2 ounces of butter
- Tbsp. of balsamic vinegar
- 3 ounces of spinach (use baby spinach)

Directions:

1. Preheat oven to 400°F
2. Put goat cheese in a baking dish that is greased. Bake 10 min.
3. Toast pumpkin seeds in a frying pan that is dry. The temperature should be reasonably high.
4. They need some color, and they should start to pop. Lower heat. Add butter and simmer till it smells nutty and is golden brown.
5. Add vinegar and boil for 3 min. Turn off heat. Spread the spinach on your plate and top with cheese and sauce.

Nutritional: Calories 824 - Fats 73 g - Carbs 3 g - Proteins 37 g

129. KORMA CURRY

Prep Time: 10 min   **Cooking Time:** 25 min   **Servings:** 6

Ingredients:

- 3-pound chicken breast, skinless, boneless
- 1 tsp. garam masala
- 1 tsp. curry powder
- 1 tbsp. apple cider vinegar
- ½ coconut cream
- 1 cup organic almond milk
- 1 tsp. ground coriander
- ¾ tsp. ground cardamom
- ½ tsp. ginger powder
- ¼ tsp. cayenne pepper
- ¾ tsp. ground cinnamon
- 1 tomato, diced
- 1 tsp. avocado oil
- ½ cup of water.

Directions:

1. Chop the chicken breast and put it in the saucepan.
2. Add avocado oil and start to cook it over medium heat.
3. Sprinkle the chicken with garam masala, curry powder, apple cider vinegar, ground coriander, cardamom, ginger powder, cayenne pepper, ground cinnamon, and diced tomato. Mix up the ingredients carefully.
4. Cook them for 10 min.
5. Add water, coconut cream, and almond milk. Sauté the meat for 10 min. more.

Nutrition: Calories: 440 kcal Fat: 32 g Fiber: 4 g Carbs: 28 g Protein: 8 g.

130. CREAMY ZOODLES

Prep Time: 15 min   **Cooking Time:** 10 min   **Servings:** 4

Ingredients:

- 1¼ cups heavy whipping cream
- ¼ cup mayonnaise
- Salt and ground black pepper, as required
- 30 oz. zucchini, spiralized with blade C
- 3 oz. Parmesan cheese, grated
- 2 tbsp. fresh mint leaves
- 2 tbsp. butter, melted

Directions:

1. The heavy cream must be added to a pan then bring to a boil.
2. Lower the heat to low and cook until reduced in half. Put in the pepper, mayo, and salt; cook until mixture is warm enough.
3. Add the zucchini noodles and gently stir to combine. Stir in the Parmesan cheese.
4. Divide the zucchini noodles onto four serving plates and immediately drizzle with the melted butter. Serve immediately.

Nutrition: Calories: 241 kcal Fat: 11.4 g Fiber: 7.5 g Carbs: 3.1 g Protein: 5.1 g.

131. CHEESY BACON SQUASH SPAGHETTI

Prep Time: 30 min   **Cooking Time:** 50 min   **Servings:** 4

Ingredients:

- 2 pounds spaghetti squash
- 2 pounds bacon
- ½ cup of butter
- 2 cups of shredded parmesan cheese
- Salt
- Black pepper.

Directions:

1. Let the oven preheat to 375°F.
2. Trim or remove each stem of spaghetti squash, slice into rings no more than an inch wide, and take out the seeds. Lay the sliced rings down on the baking sheet, bake for 40-45 min.
3. It is ready when the strands separate easily when a fork is used to scrape it. Let it cool.
4. Cook sliced up bacon until crispy. Take out and let it cool. Take off the shell on each ring, separate each strand with a fork, and put them in a bowl. Heat the strands in a microwave to get them warm, then put in butter and stir around till the butter melts.
5. Pour in parmesan cheese and bacon crumbles and add salt and pepper to your taste. Enjoy.

Nutrition: Calories: 398 kcal Fat: 12.5 g Fiber: 9.4 g Carbs: 4.1 g Protein: 5.1 g.

132. PORTOBELLO STUFFED MUSHROOMS

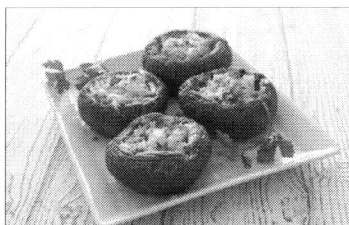

Prep Time: 10 min   **Cooking Time**:10 min   **Servings**: 4

Ingredients:

- 2 2 oz. artichoke hearts, drained, chopped
- 1 tbsp. coconut cream
- 1 tbsp. cream cheese
- 1 tsp. minced garlic
- 1 tbsp. fresh cilantro, chopped
- 3 oz. Cheddar cheese, grated
- ½ tsp. ground black pepper
- 2 tbsp. olive oil
- ½ tsp. salt.

portobello mushrooms

- 1 cup spinach, chopped, steamed

Directions:

1. Sprinkle mushrooms with olive oil and place in the tray. Transfer the tray to the preheated to 360°F oven and broil them for 5 min.
2. Meanwhile, blend artichoke hearts, coconut cream, cream cheese, minced garlic, and chopped cilantro.
3. Add grated cheese to the mixture and sprinkle with ground black pepper and salt.
4. Fill the broiled mushrooms with the cheese mixture and cook them for 5 min. more. Serve the mushrooms only hot.

Nutrition: Calories: 135.2 kcal Total Fat: 5.5 g Cholesterol: 16.4 mg Sodium: 698.1 mg Potassium: 275.3 mg Carbs: 8.4g Protein: 14.8 g.

133. BRUSSELS SPROUTS WITH BACON

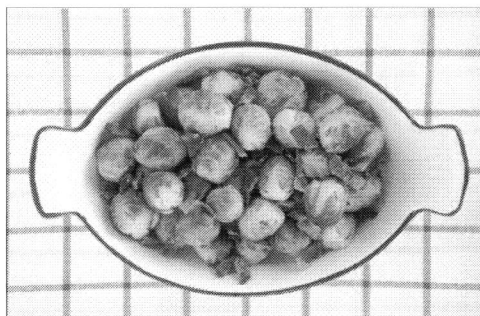

Prep Time: 15 min   **Cooking Time**: 40 min   **Servings**: 6

Ingredients:

- 16 oz. bacon
- 16 oz. Brussel sprouts
- Black pepper.

Directions:

1. Warm the oven to reach 400°F.
2. Slice the bacon into small lengthwise pieces. Put the sprouts and bacon with pepper.
3. Bake within 35 to 40 min. Serve.

Nutrition: Calories: 113 kcal Carbs: 3.9 g Protein: 7.9 g Total Fats: 6.9 g.

134. MUSHROOM OMELET

Prep. Time: 5 Min.   **Cooking Time**: 10 Min.   **Servings**: 1

Ingredients:

- 4 sliced large mushrooms
- A quarter chopped yellow onion
- A single ounce of shredded cheese
- An ounce of butter
- 3 eggs

Directions:

1. Crack the eggs and whisk them.
2. When smooth and frothy, they are right.
3. Melt butter over medium heat in a frying pan.
4. Add onions and mushrooms and stir until they become tender. Pour the egg mix in. Surround the veggies.
5. When the omelet begins to get firm but is still a little raw on top, add cheese.
6. Carefully ease around the edges and fold in half.
7. When it's golden-brown underneath (turning this color), remove and plate it.

Nutrition: Calories 517 - Fats 4 g - Carbs 5 g - Proteins 26 g

135. TUNA CASSEROLE

Prep. Time: 7 Min.   **Cooking Time**: 20 Min.   **Servings**: 4

Ingredients:

- A single green bell pepper
- 5 ⅓ celery stalks
- 16 ounces of tuna in olive oil and drained
- A single yellow onion
- 2 ounces of butter
- A single cup of mayo
- 4 ounces of parmesan cheese freshly shredded
- A single tsp. of chili flakes

Directions:

1. Preheat your oven to 400°F
2. Chop all of the bell peppers, onions, and celery finely before frying it in butter in a frying pan. They should be slightly soft.
3. Mix mayo and tuna with flakes and cheese.
4. This should be done in a greased baking dish.
5. Add the veggies.
6. Stir.
7. Bake 20 min.
8. It should be golden brown.

Nutrition: Calories 653 - Fats 43 g - Proteins 23 g - Carbs 5 g

136. GOAT CHEESE FRITTATA

Prep. Time: 15 Min.   **Cooking Time**: 30 Min.   **Servings**: 2

Ingredients:

- 4 ounces of goat cheese
- 5 ounces of mushrooms
- 3 ounces of fresh spinach
- 2 ounces of scallions
- 2 ounces of butter
- Half a dozen eggs

Directions:

1. Preheat your oven to 350°F
2. Crack the eggs and whisk before crumbling cheese in the mix. Cut mushrooms into wedge shapes. Chop up the scallions.
3. Melt the butter in a skillet that is oven-proof and cook scallions and mushrooms over medium heat for 10 min. They will be golden brown (or should be).
4. Add spinach and sauté for two min.
5. Pour egg mixture into the skillet.
6. Place in the oven uncovered and bake for 20 min.
7. It should be golden brown in the center.

Nutritional: Calories 774 - Fats 67 g - Carbs 6 g - Proteins 35 g

137. KETO PASTA

Prep. Time: 5 Min.   **Cooking Time**: 1 Min.   **Servings**: 1

Ingredients:

- A single large egg yolk
- A single cup of mozzarella cheese that is part-skim low moisture and shredded

Directions:

1. In a bowl safe for the microwave, you will need to microwave the cheese for 60 seconds.
2. Stir until it's melted. Allow cooling for 60 seconds. Add in yolk and stir. It should make a yellow dough. Place it on a flat surface that has been lined with parchment paper.
3. Place another paper over the dough.
4. Get a rolling pin and roll dough.
5. Remove the top piece when the dough is an eighth of an inch thick. Cut the dough into half-inch wide strips. Put in the fridge for 6 hours. Put pasta in a pot of boiling water to cook and do not add salt.
6. Cook for 60 seconds, don't cook too long.
7. Remove and run under cold water.
8. Separate the strands.

Nutrition: Calories 358 - Fats 22 g - Carbs 3 g - Proteins 33 g

138.   MEATY SALAD

Prep. Time: 5 Min.   **Cooking Time**: 10 Min.   **Servings**: 2

Ingredients:

- ounces of salami slices
- 2 cups of spinach
- A single avocado large and diced
- 2 tbsp. of olive oil
- A single tsp. of balsamic vinegar

Directions:

1. Toss it all together.

Nutrition: Calories 454 - Fats 42 g - Carbs 10 g - Proteins 9 g

139.   TOMATO SALAD

Prep. Time: 10 Min   **Cooking Time**: 5 Min.   **Servings**: 2

Ingredients:

- A dozen small spear asparagus
- 4 raw cherry tomatoes
- A cup and a half of arugula
- A single tbsp. of olive oil
- A tbsp. of whole pieces' pine nuts
- A tsp. of maple syrup
- Tbsp. balsamic vinegar
- 2 tbsp. soft goat cheese

Directions:

2. Cut the tough ends off asparagus and throw them away. Place the asparagus in a pan of boiling water and cook for 3 min.
3. Put in a bowl of ice-cold water right away.
4. Chill for 60 seconds. Drain. Put on a plate.
5. Slice your tomatoes in half, place them on top of the greens. (Arugula and asparagus)
6. Toss to combine.
7. Add the nuts to a pan that's dry and on a low heat toast for 2 min. until it is lightly golden.
8. Add the syrup and vinegar along with the olive oil to a bowl and whisk, so they combine.
9. Drizzle the dressing on top and crumble your cheese.
10. Sprinkle the nuts over the top.

Nutrition: Calories 234 - Fats 18 g - Carbs 7 g - Proteins 7 g

140.   KALUA PORK WITH CABBAGE

Prep Time: 10 min   **Cooking Time**: 8 h   **Servings**: 4

Ingredients:

- 1-pound boneless pork butt roast
- Pink Himalayan salt
- Freshly ground black pepper
- 1 tbsp. smoked paprika or Liquid Smoke
- ½ cup of water
- ½ head cabbage, chopped.

Directions:

1. With the crock insert in place, preheat the slow cooker to low. Generously season the pork roast with pink Himalayan salt, pepper, and smoked paprika. Place the pork roast in the slow-cooker insert, and add the water.
2. Cover and cook on low for 7 hours.
3. Transfer the cooked pork roast to a plate. Put the chopped cabbage in the bottom of the slow cooker, and put the pork roast back in on the cabbage.
4. Cover and cook the cabbage and pork roast for 1 hour.
5. Remove the pork roast from the slow cooker and place it on a baking sheet. Use two forks to shred the pork. Serve the shredded pork hot with the cooked cabbage.

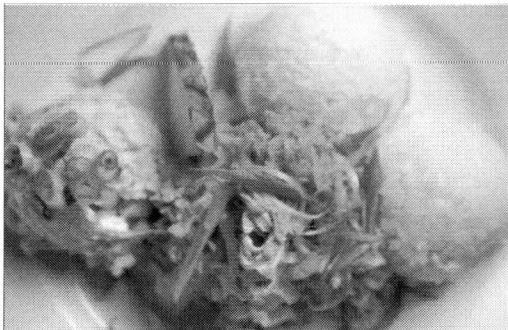

6. Reserve the liquid from the slow cooker to remoisten the pork and cabbage when reheating leftovers.

Nutrition: Calories: 451 kcal | Fat: 19.3 g | Carbs: 2.1 g | Fiber: 11.2 g | Protein: 14.3 g.

141. COFFEE BBQ PORK BELLY

Prep Time: 15 min   **Cooking Time**: 60 min   **Servings**: 4

Ingredients:

- 1½ cup beef stock
- 2 lb. pork belly
- 4 tbsp. olive oil
- Low-carb barbecue dry rub
- 2 tbsp. instant Espresso Powder.

Directions:

1. Set the oven at 350°F. Heat-up the beef stock in a small saucepan.
2. Mix in the dry barbecue rub and espresso powder. Put the pork belly, skin side up in a shallow dish and drizzle half of the oil over the top.
3. Put the hot stock around the pork belly. Bake within 45 min.
4. Sear each slice within three min. per side. Serve.

Nutrition: Calories: 644 kcal Carbs: 2.6 g Protein: 24 g Total Fats: 68 g.

142. GARLIC & THYME LAMB CHOPS

Prep Time: 15 min   **Cooking Time:** 10 min   **Servings**: 6

Ingredients:

- 6 - 4 oz. lamb chops
- 4 whole garlic cloves
- 2 thyme sprigs
- 1 tsp. ground thyme
- 3 tbsp. olive oil.

Directions:

1. Warm-up a skillet. Put the olive oil. Rub the chops with the spices.
2. Put the chops in the skillet with the garlic and sprigs of thyme.
3. Sauté within 3 to 4 min. and serve.

Nutrition: Calories: 252 kcal Carbs: 1 g Protein: 14 g Fats: 21 g.

143. LEMON FISH

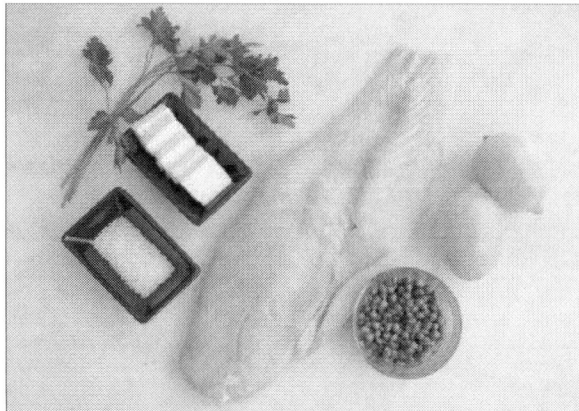

Prep. Time: 10 Min.   **Cooking Time**: 20 Min.

Servings: 6

Ingredients:

- 1 tbsp. lemon juice
- 4 tbsp. butter, unsalted
- Sea salt & pepper, to taste
- 2 tbsp. almond flour
- 2 tbsp. olive oil
- 2 tilapia fillets
- Sea salt & pepper, to taste

Directions:

1. Warm the butter in a small pan over medium heat. Warm the butter until it's slightly browned. Add the lemon juice, pepper, and salt and stir constantly. Adjust seasoning to taste.
2. Set aside while you cook your fillets.
3. Rinse the fish fillets and pat them dry before sprinkling them with salt and pepper.
4. Spread the flour on a plate or shallow dish and dredge the fillets, spreading the flour over the fillets as needed. Heat a non-stick skillet over medium heat and warm the oil in it until it's shimmering.
5. Place the fillets in the pan and cook for about

two min. per side until golden and crisp on either side.

6. Remove the fish from the heat and place it on the plate.

7. Drizzle the sauce over it and serve immediately!

Nutrition: Calories 393 - Fats 28 g - Carbs 3 g - Proteins 31

144. JAMAICAN JERK PORK ROAST

Prep Time: 15 min   **Cooking Time:** 4 h   **Servings:** 12

Ingredients:

- 1 tbsp. olive oil
- 4 lb. pork shoulder
- ½ cup beef Broth
- ¼ cup Jamaican Jerk spice blend.

Directions:

1. Rub the roast well the oil and the jerk spice blend.
2. Sear the roast on all sides.
3. Put the beef broth.
4. Simmer within 4 hours on low.
5. Shred and serve.

Nutrition: Calories: 282 kcal Carbs: 0 g Protein: 23 g Fats: 20 g.

145. KETO MEATBALLS

Prep Time: 15 min   **Cooking Time:** 20 min   **Servings:** 10

Ingredients:

- 1 egg
- ½ cup grated parmesan
- ½ cup shredded mozzarella
- 1 lb. ground beef
- 1 tbsp. garlic.

Directions:

1. Warm-up the oven to reach 400°F.
2. Combine all of the fixings. Shape into meatballs.
3. Bake within 18-20 min.
4. Cool and serve.

Nutrition: Calories: 153 kcal Carbs: 0.7 g Protein: 12.2 g Fats: 10.9 g.

146. MIXED VEGETABLE PATTIES

Prep Time: 15 min   **Cooking Time:** 10 min   **Servings:** 4

Ingredients:

- 1 cup cauliflower florets
- 1 bag vegetables
- 1½ cup Water
- 1 cup flax meal
- 2 tbsp. olive oil.

Directions:

1. Steam the veggies to the steamer basket within 4 to 5 min.
2. Mash in the flax meal.
3. Shape into 4 patties.
4. Cook the patties within 3 min. per side. Serve.

Nutrition: Calories: 220 kcal Carbs: 3 g Protein: 4 g Fats: 10 g.

147. ROASTED LEG OF LAMB

Prep Time: 15 min   **Cooking Time:** 1 h 30 min   **Servings:** 6

Ingredients:

- ½ cup reduced-sodium beef broth
- 2 lb. lamb leg
- 6 garlic cloves
- 1 tbsp. rosemary leaves
- 1 tsp. black pepper.

Directions:

1. Warm-up oven temperature to 400°F.
2. Put the lamb in the pan and put the broth and seasonings.
3. Roast 30 min. and lower the heat to 350°F. Cook within 1 hour.
4. Cool and serve.

Nutrition: Calories: 223 kcal Carbs: 1 g Protein: 22 g Fats: 14 g.

148. MONGOLIAN BEEF

Prep Time: 15 min   **Cooking Time**: 10 min   **Servings**: 4

Ingredients:

- 1 lb. grass-fed flank steak, cut into thin slices against the grain
- 2 tsp. arrowroot starch
- Salt, to taste
- ¼ cup avocado oil
- 1 (1-inch) piece fresh ginger, grated
- 4 garlic cloves, minced
- ½ tsp. red pepper flakes, crushed
- ¼ cup water
- ⅓ cup low-sodium soy sauce
- 1 tsp. red boat fish sauce
- 3 scallions, sliced
- 1 tsp. sesame seeds.

Direction:

1. In a bowl, add the steak slices, arrowroot starch, salt, and toss to coat well.
2. In a larger skillet, heat oil over medium-high heat and cook the steak slices for about 1½ min. per side.
3. With a slotted spoon, transfer the steak slices onto a plate.
4. Drain the oil from the skillet but leaving about 1 tbsp. inside.
5. In the same skillet, add the ginger, garlic, red pepper flakes, and sauté for about 1 min.
6. Add the water, soy sauce, fish sauce, and stir to combine well. Stir in the cooked steak slices and simmer for about 3 min.
7. Stir in the scallions and simmer for about 2 min.
8. Remove from the heat and serve hot with the garnishing of sesame seeds.

Nutrition: Calories: 266 kcal Carbs: 5.7 g Sugar: 1.7 g Fiber: 1.2 g Protein: 34 g Fat: 11.7 g Sodium: 1350 mg.

149. LETTUCE SALAD

Prep Time: 10 min   **Cooking Time**: 0 min   **Servings**: 1

Ingredients:

- 1 cup Romaine lettuce, roughly chopped
- 3 oz. seitan, chopped
- 1 tbsp. avocado oil
- 1 tsp. sunflower seeds
- 1 tsp. lemon juice
- 1 egg, boiled, peeled
- 2 oz. Cheddar cheese, shredded.

Directions:

1. Place lettuce in the salad bowl. Add chopped seitan and shredded cheese.
2. Then chop the egg roughly and add in the salad bowl too.
3. Mix up together lemon juice with the avocado oil.
4. Sprinkle the salad with the oil mixture and sunflower seeds. Don't stir the salad before serving.

Nutrition: Calories: 20 kcal Fat: 0.2 g Cholesterol: 0 mg Sodium: 31 mg Potassium: 241 mg Carbs: 4.2 g Protein: 1.2 g.

150. CHILI LIME COD

Prep. Time: 10 Min.   **Cooking Time:** 10 Min.   **Servings:** 2

Ingredients:

- 1/3 c. coconut flour
- ½ tsp. cayenne pepper
- 1 egg, beaten
- 1 lime
- 1 tsp. crushed red pepper flakes
- 1 tsp. garlic powder
- 12 oz. cod fillets
- Sea salt & pepper, to taste

Directions:

1. Preheat the oven to 400°F and line a baking sheet with non-stick foil. Place the flour in a shallow dish (a plate works fine) and drag the fillets of cod through the beaten egg.
2. Dredge the cod in the coconut flour, then lay it on the baking sheet.
3. Sprinkle the tops of the fillets with seasoning and lime juice.
4. Bake for 10 to 12 min. until the fillets are flaky.
5. Serve immediately!

Nutrition: Calories 215 - Fats 5 g - Carbs 3 g - Proteins 37 g

151. LEMON GARLIC SHRIMP PASTA

Prep. Time: 10 min.   **Cooking:** 10 min.   **Servings:** 4

Ingredients:

- ½ lemon, thinly sliced
- ½ tsp. paprika
- 1 lb. shrimp, deveined & peeled
- 1 tsp. basil, fresh & chopped
- 14 oz. Miracle Noodle Angel Hair pasta
- 2 cloves garlic, minced
- 2 tbsp. butter
- 2 tbsp. extra virgin olive oil
- Sea salt & pepper, to taste

Directions:

1. Drain the packages of Miracle noodles and rinse them under cold running water.
2. Bring a pot of water to a boil and place the noodles in the boiling water for two min. before pulling them back out again.
3. Place the boiled noodles in a hot pan over medium heat and allow the excess moisture to cook off of them. Set aside.
4. Add the butter and olive oil to the pan, then add the garlic and stir.
5. Place the shrimp and the lemon slices in the pan and allow to cook until the shrimp is done, about three min. per side.
6. Once the shrimp is done, add the salt, pepper, and paprika to the pan, then top with the noodles. Toss to coat everything together, top with basil, and serve!

Nutritional: Calories 360 - Fats 21 g - Carbs 4 g - Proteins 36 g

152. ONE-PAN TEX MEX

Prep. Time: 5 min.   **Cooking time:** 10 min.   **Servings:** 4

Ingredients:

- 1/3 c. baby corn, canned
- 1/3 c. cilantro, chopped & separated
- ½ c. chicken stock
- ½ c. diced tomatoes & green chiles
- ½ tsp. garlic powder
- ½ tsp. oregano
- 1 tsp. cumin
- 2 c. cauliflower, riced
- 2 c. chicken breast, cooked & diced

- 2 c. Mexican cheese blend, shredded
- 2 tbsp. extra virgin olive oil
- 2 tsp. chili powder

Directions:

1. Slice baby corn into small pieces and set aside.
2. Press any liquid out of the riced cauliflower and set aside. In a large pan over medium heat, warm your oil and sauté the cauliflower rice for about two min.
3. Add all ingredients except for the cheese and cilantro, and stir well to cook.
4. Stir in about half of the cilantro and allow the flavors to meld.
5. Stir about half the cheese into the mix and stir until melted and combined.
6. Serve and top with remaining cheese and cilantro for garnish!

Nutrition: Calories 345 - Fats 26 g - Carbs 7 g - Proteins 38 g

---

153. SPINACH ARTICHOKE-STUFFED CHICKEN BREASTS

Prep. Time: 15 Min. **Cooking Time:** 15 Min. **Servings:** 6

Ingredients:

- ¼ c. Greek yogurt
- ¼ c. spinach, thawed & drained
- ½ c. artichoke hearts, thinly sliced
- ½ c. mozzarella cheese, shredded
- 1 ½ lb. chicken breasts
- 2 tbsp. olive oil
- 4 oz. cream cheese
- Sea salt & pepper, to taste

Directions:

1. Pound the chicken breasts to a thickness of about one inch. Using a sharp knife, slice a "pocket" into the side of each.
2. This is where you will put the filling.
3. Sprinkle the breasts with salt and pepper and set aside.
4. In a medium bowl, combine cream cheese, yogurt, mozzarella, spinach, artichoke, salt, and pepper and mix completely.
5. A hand mixer may be the easiest way to combine all the ingredients thoroughly.
6. Spoon the mixture into each breast's pockets and set aside while you heat a large skillet over medium heat and warm the oil in it. If you have an extra filling you can't fit into the breasts, set it aside until just before your chicken is done cooking.
7. Cook each breast for about eight min. per side, then pull off the heat when it reaches an internal temperature of about 165°F.
8. Before you pull the chicken out of the pan, heat the remaining filling to warm it through and rid it of any cross-contamination from the chicken.
9. Once hot, top the chicken breasts with it.
10. Serve.

Nutritional: Calories 288 - Fats 17 g - Carbs 2 g - Proteins 28 g

---

154. CHICKEN PARMESAN

Prep. Time: 20 Min. **Cooking Time:** 15 Min. **Servings:** 4

Ingredients:

- ¼ c. avocado oil
- ¼ c. almond flour
- ¼ c. parmesan cheese, grated
- ¾ c. marinara sauce, sugar-free
- ¾ c. mozzarella cheese, shredded
- 2 lg. eggs, beaten
- 2 tsp. Italian seasoning
- 3 oz. pork rinds, pulverized
- 4 lg. chicken breasts, boneless & skinless
- Sea salt & pepper, to taste

Directions:

1. Preheat the oven to 450°F and grease a baking dish. Place the beaten egg into one shallow dish. Place the almond flour in another. In a third dish, combine the pork rinds, parmesan, and Italian seasoning and mix well.

2. Pat the chicken breasts dry and pound them down to about ½ thick.

3. Dredge the chicken in the almond flour, then coat in egg, then coat in the crumb.

4. Heat a large sauté pan over medium-high heat and warm oil until shimmering.

5. Once the oil is hot, lay the breasts into the pan and not move them until they've had a chance to cook.

6. Cook for about two min., then flip as gently as possible (a fish spatula is perfect) then cook for two more. Remove the pan from the heat.

7. Place the breasts in the greased baking dish and top with marinara sauce and mozzarella cheese.

8. Bake for about 10 min. Serve!

Nutrition: Calories 621 - Fats 34 g - Carbs 6 g - Proteins 67 g

155. GRAIN-FREE CREAMY NOODLES

Prep Time: 15 min   **Cooking Time**: 10 min   **Servings**: 4

Ingredients:

- 1¼ cup heavy whipping cream
- ¼ cup mayonnaise
- Salt and freshly ground black pepper, to taste
- 30 oz. zucchini, spiralized with blade
- 4 organic egg yolks
- 3 oz. Parmesan cheese, grated
- 2 tbsp. fresh parsley, chopped
- 2 tbsp. butter, melted.

Direction:

1. In a pan, add the heavy cream and bring to a boil.
2. Reduce the heat to low and cook until reduced.
3. Add the mayonnaise, salt, black pepper, and cook until the mixture is warm enough.
4. Add the zucchini noodles and gently, stir to combine.
5. Immediately, remove from the heat.
6. Place the zucchini noodles mixture onto 4 serving plates evenly and immediately, top with the egg yolks, followed by the parmesan and parsley.
7. Drizzle with hot melted butter and serve.

Nutrition: Calories: 427 kcal Carbs: 9 g Sugar: 3.8 g Fiber: 2.4 g Protein: 13 g Fat: 39.1 g Sodium: 412 mg.

156. MEAT-FREE ZOODLES STROGANOFF

Prep Time: 20 min   **Cooking Time**: 12 min   **Servings**: 5

Ingredients:

For Mushroom Sauce:

- 1½ tbsp. butter
- 1 large garlic clove, minced
- 1¼ cup fresh button mushrooms, sliced
- ¼ cup homemade vegetable broth
- ¼ cup cream
- Salt and freshly ground black pepper, to taste.

For Zucchini Noodles:

- 3 large zucchinis, spiralized with blade
- ¼ cup fresh parsley leaves, chopped.

Direction:

1. For mushroom sauce: in a large skillet, melt the butter over medium heat and sauté the garlic for about 1 min.
2. Stir in the mushrooms and cook for about 6-8 min.
3. Stir in the broth and cook for about 2 min., stirring continuously.
4. Stir in the cream, salt, and black pepper and cook for about 1 min.

5. Meanwhile, for the zucchini noodles: in a large pan of boiling water, add the zucchini noodles and cook for about 2-3 min.

6. With a slotted spoon, transfer the zucchini noodles into a colander and immediately rinse under cold running water.

7. Drain the zucchini noodles well and transfer onto a large paper towel-lined plate to drain.

8. Divide the zucchini noodles onto serving plates evenly.

9. Remove the mushroom sauce from the heat and place over zucchini noodles evenly.

10. Serve immediately with the garnishing of parsley.

Nutrition: Calories: 77 kcal Carbs: 7.9 g Sugar: 4 g Fiber: 2.4 g Protein: 3.4 g Fat: 4.6 g Sodium: 120 mg.

157. EYE-CATCHING VEGGIES

Prep Time: 51 min **Cooking Time:** 20 min **Servings:** 4

Ingredients:

- ¼ cup butter
- 6 scallions, sliced
- 1 lb. fresh white mushrooms, sliced
- 1 cup tomatoes, crushed
- Salt and freshly ground black pepper, to taste
- 2 tbsp. feta cheese, crumbled

Direction:

1. In a large pan, melt the butter over medium-low heat and sauté the scallion for about 2 min.

2. Add the mushrooms and sauté for about 5-7 min.

3. Stir in the tomatoes and cook for about 8-10 min., stirring occasionally.

4. Stir in the salt and black pepper and remove from the heat.

5. Serve with the topping of feta.

Nutrition: Calories: 160 kcal Carbs: 7.4 g Sugar: 3.9 g Fiber: 2.3 g Protein: 5.5 g Fat: 13.5 g Sodium: 211 mg.

158. CHICKEN SCHNITZEL

Prep Time: 15 min **Cooking Time:** 15-22 min **Servings:** 4

Ingredients:

- 1 tbsp. chopped fresh parsley
- 4 garlic cloves, minced
- 1 tbsp. plain vinegar
- 1 tbsp. coconut aminos
- 2 tsp. sugar-free maple syrup
- 2 tsp. chili pepper
- Salt and black pepper to taste
- 6 tbsp. coconut oil
- 1 lb. asparagus, hard stems removed
- 4 chicken breasts, skin-on and boneless
- 2 cups grated Mexican cheese blend
- 1 tbsp. mixed sesame seeds
- 1 cup almond flour
- 4 eggs, beaten
- 6 tbsp. avocado oil
- 1 tsp. chili flakes for garnish

Directions:

1. In a bowl, whisk the parsley, garlic, vinegar, coconut aminos, maple syrup, chili pepper, salt, and black pepper. Set aside.

2. Heat the coconut oil in a large skillet and stir-fry the asparagus for 8 to 10 min. or until tender. Remove the asparagus into a large bowl and toss with the vinegar mixture. Set aside for serving. Cover the chicken breasts in plastic wraps and use a meat tenderizer to pound the chicken until flattened to 2-inch thickness gently.

3. On a plate, mix the Mexican cheese blend and sesame seeds. Dredge the chicken pieces in the almond flour, dip in the egg on both sides, and generously coat in the seed mix.

4. Heat the avocado oil. Cook the chicken until golden brown and cooked within.

5. Divide the asparagus onto four serving plates, place a chicken on each, and garnish with the chili flakes. Serve warm.

Nutrition: Calories: 451 kcal Fat: 18.5 g Carbs: 5.9 g Fiber: 12.9 g Protein: 19.5 g.

159. CHICKEN ROLLATINI

Prep Time: 15 min   **Cooking Time:** 30 min   **Servings:** 4

Ingredients:

- 4 (3-ounce) boneless skinless chicken breasts, pounded to about 1/3-inch thick
- 4 oz. ricotta cheese
- 4 slices prosciutto (4 oz)
- 1 cup fresh spinach
- ½ cup almond flour
- ½ cup grated Parmesan cheese
- 2 eggs, beaten
- ¼ cup good-quality olive oil.

Directions:

1. Preheat the oven. Set the oven temperature to 400°F.
2. Prepare the chicken—Pat the chicken breasts dry with paper towels. Spread ¼ of the ricotta in the middle of each breast.
3. Place the prosciutto over the ricotta and ¼ cup of the spinach on the prosciutto.
4. Fold the long edges of the chicken breast over the filling, then roll the chicken breast up to enclose the filling.
5. Place the rolls seam-side down on your work surface.
6. Bread the chicken. On a plate, stir together the almond flour and Parmesan and set it next to the beaten eggs.
7. Carefully dip a chicken roll in the egg, then roll it in the almond-flour mixture until it is completely covered.
8. Set the rolls seam-side down on your work surface. Repeat with the other rolls.
9. Brown the rolls. In a medium skillet over medium heat, warm the olive oil.
10. Place the rolls seam-side down in the skillet and brown them on all sides, turning them carefully, about 10 min.in total.
11. Transfer the rolls, seam-side down, to a 9-by-9-inch baking dish—Bake the chicken rolls for 25 min., or until they're cooked through.
12. Serve. Place one chicken roll on each of four plates and serve them immediately.

Nutrition: Calories: 365 kcal Fat: 17.1 g Fiber: 9.4 g Carbs: 3.2 g Protein: 1.4 g.

160. LOW CARB BROCCOLI MASH

Prep Time: 10 min   **Cooking Time:** 5 min   **Servings:** 2

Ingredients:

- 12 oz. broccoli
- ½ clove garlic
- 2 tbsp. parsley
- Salt, to taste
- 1½ oz. butter
- Pepper, to taste.

Directions:

1. Put salt into the water and boil. Put broccoli florets and cook within a few min. Remove the water and separate the soft broccoli.
2. Place all fixing in a blender and pulse. Serve.

Nutrition: Calories: 210 kcal Fats: 18 g Carbs: 7 g Fiber: 18 g Proteins: 5 g.

161. AVOCADO LOW CARB BURGER

Prep Time: 15 min   **Cooking Time**: 25 min   **Servings:** 4

Ingredients:

- 1 avocado
- 1 leaf lettuce
- 2 slices of prosciutto or any ham
- 1 slice of tomato
- 1 egg
- ½ tbsp. olive oil for frying.

For the sauce:

- 1 tbsp. low carb mayonnaise
- ¼ tsp. low carb hot sauce
- ¼ tsp. mustard
- ¼ tsp. Italian seasoning
- ½ tsp. sesame seeds (optional).

Directions:

1. In a small bowl, combine keto-friendly mayonnaise, mustard, hot sauce, and Italian seasoning.
2. Heat 1/2 tbsp. of olive oil in a pan and cook an egg. The yolk must be fluid.
3. Cut the avocado in half, remove the peel and bone. Cut the narrowest part of the avocado so that the fruit can stand on a plate.
4. Fill the hole in one half of the avocado with the prepared sauce.
5. Top with lettuce, prosciutto strips, a slice of tomato, and a fried egg.
6. Cover with the other half of the avocado and sprinkle with sesame seeds (optional).

Nutrition: Calories: 416 kcal Carbs: 15 g Fat: 24 g Protein: 35 g.

162. INCREDIBLE SALMON DISH

Prep Time: 10 min **Cooking Time:** 15 min **Servings:** 4

Ingredients:

- 3 cups of ice water
- 2 tsp. sriracha sauce
- 4 tsp. stevia
- 3 scallions, chopped
- Black pepper and salt to taste
- 2 tsp. flaxseed oil
- 4 tsp. apple cider vinegar
- 3 tsp. avocado oil
- 4 medium salmon fillets
- 4 cups baby arugula
- 2 cups cabbage, finely chopped
- 1½ tsp. Jamaican jerk seasoning
- ¼ cup pepitas, toasted
- 2 cups watermelon radish, julienned.

Directions:

1. Put ice water in a bowl, add scallions and leave aside.
2. In another bowl, mix sriracha sauce with stevia and stir well.
3. Transfer 2 tsp. of this mix to a bowl and mix with half of the avocado oil, flaxseed oil, vinegar, salt and pepper, and whisk.
4. Sprinkle jerk seasoning over salmon, rub with sriracha and stevia mix and season with salt and pepper.
5. Heat-up a pan with the rest of the avocado oil over medium-high heat, add salmon, flesh side down, cook for 4 min., flip and cook for 4 min. more and divide among plates.
6. In a bowl, mix radishes with cabbage and arugula.
7. Add salt, pepper, sriracha and vinegar mix and toss well.
8. Add this to salmon fillets, drizzle the remaining sriracha and stevia sauce all over and top with pepitas and drained scallions. Enjoy!

Nutrition: Calories: 160 kcal Fat: 6 g Carbs: 1 g Fiber: 1 g Protein: 12 g.

163. CHICKEN PARMESAN

Prep. Time: 20 Min. **Cooking Time:** 15 Min. **Servings:** 4

Ingredients:

- ¼ c. avocado oil
- ¼ c. almond flour
- ¼ c. parmesan cheese, grated
- ¾ c. marinara sauce, sugar-free
- ¾ c. mozzarella cheese, shredded
- 2 lg. eggs, beaten
- 2 tsp. Italian seasoning
- 3 oz. pork rinds, pulverized
- 4 lg. chicken breasts, boneless & skinless
- Sea salt & pepper, to taste

Directions:

1. Preheat the oven to 450°F and grease a baking dish.
2. Place the beaten egg into one shallow dish. Place the almond flour in another. In a third dish, combine the pork rinds, parmesan, and Italian seasoning and mix well.
3. Pat the chicken breasts dry and pound them down to about ½ thick.

4. Dredge the chicken in the almond flour, then coat in egg, then coat in the crumb.

5. Heat a large sauté pan over medium-high heat and warm oil until shimmering.

6. Once the oil is hot, lay the breasts into the pan and not move them until they've had a chance to cook.

7. Cook for about two min., then flip as gently as possible (a fish spatula is perfect) then cook for two more. Remove the pan from the heat.

8. Place the breasts in the greased baking dish and top with marinara sauce and mozzarella cheese.

9. Bake for about 10 min.

10. Serve!

Nutrition: Calories 621 Fats 34 g Carbs 6 g Proteins 67 g

164.   HEARTY LUNCH SALAD WITH BROCCOLI AND BACON

Prep. Time: 10 Min.   **Cooking Time**: 10 Min.   **Servings**: 5

Ingredients:

- 4 cups broccoli florets, chopped
- 7 slices bacon, fried and crumbled
- ¼ cup red onion, diced
- ¼ cup almonds, sliced
- ½ cup mayo
- ¼ cup sour cream
- 1 tsp white distilled vinegar
- salt
- 6 oz. cheddar, cut into small cubes

Directions:

1. In a mixing bowl, combine the cheddar, broccoli, bacon, almonds, and onion.
2. Stir these ingredients thoroughly.
3. In another bowl, combine the sour cream, mayo, vinegar, and salt. Stir the ingredients well and pour this mixture over your broccoli salad.

Nutrition: Calories 267 Fats 20 g Carbs 7 g Proteins 12 g

165.   FATTY BURGER BOMBS

Prep. Time: 15 min.   **Cooking Time**: 15 min.   **Servings**: 20

Ingredients:

- 1-pound ground beef
- ½ tsp garlic powder
- Kosher salt and black pepper
- 1 oz. cold butter, cut into 20 pieces
- ½ block cheddar cheese, cut into 20 pieces

Directions:

1. Preheat the oven to 375°F.
2. In a separate bowl, then mix ground beef, garlic powder, salt, and pepper.
3. Use a mini muffin tin to form your bombs.
4. Put about 1 Tbsp. of beef into each muffin tin cup.
5. Make sure that you completely cover the bottom. Add a piece of butter on top and put 1 Tbsp. of beef over the butter.
6. Place a piece of cheese on the top and put the remaining beef over the cheese.
7. Bake your bombs for about 15 min.

Nutrition: Calories 80 Fats 7 g Carbs 0 g Proteins 5 g

166.   AVOCADO TACO

Prep. Time: 10 min.   **Cooking Time**: 15 min.   **Servings**: 6

Ingredients:

- 1-pound ground beef
- 3 avocados, halved
- 1 Tbsp. Chili powder
- ½ tsp salt
- ¾ tsp cumin
- ½ tsp oregano, dried
- ¼ tsp garlic powder
- ¼ tsp onion powder
- 8 Tbsp. tomato sauce
- 1 cup cheddar cheese, shredded
- ¼ cup cherry tomatoes, sliced
- ¼ cup lettuce, shredded
- ½ cup sour cream

Directions:

1. Pit halved avocados. Set aside.
2. Place the ground beef into a saucepan.
3. Cook over medium heat until it is browned.
4. Add the seasoning and tomato sauce.
5. Stir well and cook for about 4 min.
6. Load each avocado half with the beef.
7. Top with shredded cheese and lettuce, tomato slices, and sour cream.

Nutrition: Calories 278 Fats 22 g Carbs 2 g Proteins 18 g

---

167. CHICKEN QUESADILLAS

Prep. Time: 10 min.   **Cooking Time**: 15 min.   **Servings**: 2

Ingredients:

- 1½ cups Mozzarella cheese, shredded
- 1½ cups Cheddar cheese, shredded
- 1 cup chicken, cooked and shredded
- 1 bell pepper, sliced
- ¼ cup tomato, diced
- ⅛ cup green onion
- 1 Tbsp. extra-virgin olive oil

Directions:

1. Preheat the oven to 400°F. Use parchment paper to cover a pizza pan.
2. Combine your cheeses and bake the cheese shell for about 5 min. Put the chicken on one-half of the cheese shell.
3. Add peppers, tomatoes, green onion and fold your shell in half over the fillings.
4. Return your folded cheese shell to the oven again for 4-5 min.

Nutrition: Calories 599 Fats 40.5 g Carbs 6.1 g Proteins 52.7 g

---

168. SALMON SUSHI ROLLS

Prep. Time: 15 min.   **Cooking Time**: 15 min.   **Servings**: 5

Ingredients:

- 4 oz. smoked salmon
- ¼ red bell pepper, cut into matchstick pieces
- ½ cucumber, cut into matchstick pieces ½ cup Water
- ½ avocado
- 20 seaweed sheets

Directions:

1. Cut the salmon and avocado the same way that you cut the red pepper and cucumber.
2. Place seaweed snacks on a cutting board.
3. Put a cup of water nearby.
4. Wet your fingers with water and wet one edge of each seaweed sheet.
5. Put one piece of salmon, pepper, cucumber, and avocado on each seaweed snack and roll them up.

Nutrition: Calories 320 Fats 20 g Carbs 8 g Proteins 24 g

169. MEDITERRANEAN SALAD WITH GRILLED CHICKEN

Prep. Time: 15-30 min.   **Cooking Time:** 15 min.   **Servings:** 4

Ingredients:

- 4 romaine lettuce leaves, washed and dried
- 1 cucumber, diced
- 2 tomatoes, diced
- 1 red onion, sliced
- 1 avocado, sliced
- ⅓ cup Kalamata olives, pitted and chopped
- 2 Tbsp. olive oil
- ¼ cup lemon juice
- 2 Tbsp. water
- 2 Tbsp. red wine vinegar
- 2 Tbsp. parsley, chopped
- 2 Tbsp. basil, dried
- 2 Tbsp. garlic, chopped
- 1 tsp oregano, dried
- 1 tsp salt
- Black pepper, to taste
- 1-pound chicken fillets

Directions:

1. To make the marinade, mix the olive oil, lemon juice, water, red wine vinegar, parsley, basil, oregano, salt, and pepper. Divide the marinade into two halves.
2. Place the chicken into the marinade for 15-30 min.
3. In a separate bowl combine the lettuce leaves, cucumber, tomatoes, onion, avocado and olives. Stir well.
4. Pour 1 Tbsp. of oil into a pan and grill the chicken until it is browned on both sides. Slice your chicken and add it to the salad.
5. Sprinkle your salad with the remaining marinade.

Nutrition: Calories 336 Fats 21 g Carbs 13 g Proteins 24 g

170. CREAMY CAULIFLOWER SOUP

Prep. Time: 10 min.   **Cooking Time:** 40 min.   **Servings:** 5

Ingredients:

- 21 head cauliflower, cut into florets
- 3 Tbsp. olive oil
- ¾ tsp sea salt
- 4 cloves garlic
- 1 Tbsp. thyme, fresh
- 4 cups chicken broth
- 8 oz. cream cheese, cut into cubes
- ¼ tsp black pepper
- Green onion, chopped
- Parsley, chopped

Directions:

1. Preheat the oven to 425°F.
2. Place the cauliflower florets into a bowl.
3. 2 Tbsp. of olive oil over them and ¼ tsp of sea salt. Bake for about 30 min.in the oven.
4. Place the remaining olive oil in a pot, add the garlic and thyme and sauté for 1 min.
5. Pour the chicken broth and baked cauliflower into the pot.
6. Boil for 5-10 min.
7. Add the cream cheese and mix the soup with an immersion blender.
8. Top with green onion and parsley.

Nutrition: Calories 286 Fats 24 g Carbs 12 g Proteins 6 g

171. EGG DROP SOUP

Prep. Time: 10 min.   **Cooking Time:** 20 min.   **Servings** 6

Ingredients:

- 1 tbsp. olive oil
- 6 cups chicken broth, divided
- 1 tbsp. arrowroot powder
- Ground white pepper, to taste
- 1 tbsp. garlic, minced
- 2 organic eggs
- 1/3 cup fresh lemon juice
- ¼ cup scallion (green part), chopped

Directions:

1. In a large soup pan, heat the oil over medium-high heat and sauté garlic for about 1 min.
2. Add 5½ cups of broth and bring to a boil over high heat. Adjust the heat to medium and simmer for about 5 min. Meanwhile, in a bowl, add eggs, arrowroot powder, lemon juice, white pepper, and remaining broth, and beat until well combined.
3. Slowly, add the egg mixture to the pan, stirring continuously.
4. Simmer for about 5–6 min. or until the desired thickness of the soup, stirring continuously.
5. Serve hot with the garnishing of scallion.

Nutrition: Calories 92 - Fats 5.3 g - Carbs 3.4 g - Proteins 7 g

172. BROCCOLI CHEESE SOUP

Prep. Time: 5 min.   **Cooking Time:** 20 min.   **Servings:** 8

Ingredients:

- Broccoli (4 cups, chopped)
- Garlic (4 cloves, minced)
- Chicken broth (3.5 cups)
- Heavy cream (1 cup)
- Cheddar cheese (3 cups, shredded)

Directions:

1. Set a large greased saucepan with garlic over medium heat.
2. Sauté until fragrant (about a min.).
3. Add in your remaining ingredients except for cheese, and switch to high heat.
4. Allow to come to a boil, then switch the heat to low and allow to simmer until broccoli becomes fork-tender.
5. Gradually add cheese, while stirring, and continue to simmer until the cheese has been fully melted. Serve immediately and enjoy!

Nutrition: Calories 266 Fats 22.6 g Carbs 2.6 g Proteins 13.6 g

173. CREAMY TOMATO-BASIL SOUP

Prep. Time: 5 min.   **Cooking Time:** 15 min.   **Servings:** 4

Ingredients:

- 2 ounces cream cheese
- 1 (14.5-ounce) can diced tomatoes
- ¼ cup chopped fresh basil leaves
- ¼ cup heavy (whipping) cream
- 4 tbsp. butter

Directions:

1. In a food processor, add the tomatoes with juices and pulse until smooth.
2. In a medium saucepan, add the tomatoes, heavy cream, cream cheese, and butter over medium heat and cook for 10 min., stirring often. Stir in the basil, salt and pepper and cook for 5 min. or until smooth.
3. Pour the soup into two bowls and serve.

Nutrition: Calories 239 Fats 22 g Carbs 9 g Proteins 3 g

174.   SPICY CAULIFLOWER SOUP

Prep. Time: 10 min.   **Cooking Time**: 13 min.   **Servings**: 4

Ingredients:

- 1 1/2 cups water
- 1 cup carrot, sliced into 2-inch thick pieces
- 1 tsp. salt
- 2 cup cauliflower florets, sliced into 3 to 4-inch chunks
- 1 cup (canned) tomatoes
- 1 onion (large) sliced into 2-inch thick pieces
- 1 tsp. turmeric
- 1 to 1 1/2 tsp. Sambhar powder

Directions:

1. Put all the ingredients in the inner pot; stir to mix well. Secure the lid and place the pressure valve to seal position.
2. Set to LOW PRESSURE for 3 min.
3. NPR for 10 min.when the timer beeps and QPR; unlock the lid and open.
4. Stir to mix well.
5. Serve.

Nutrition: Calories 43 - Fats 0.3 g - Carbs 6.3 g - Proteins 2 g

175.   CHEESE & BACON CAULIFLOWER SOUP

Prep. Time: 10 min.   **Cooking Time**: 30 min.   **Servings**: 5

Ingredients:

- 1 cup celery
- 1 head cauliflower
- 1/2 stick butter
- 2 clove garlic (large)
- 3/4 cup cream (heavy)
- 1 cup cheddar cheese
- 1/2 cup parmesan, extra for garnish
- 1/3 cup carrots
- 3 bacon slices
- 32 ounces chicken stock

Directions:

1. Chop 1/2 of the cauliflower; grate the other half. Prepare the other veggies. Set the IP to SAUTÉ. Add the bacon; cook till crisped and remove.
2. Add the butter to the pot. Add the grated cauliflower. Add the rest of the veggies; sauté for 5 min. Add the cream; stir to mix.
3. Add the garlic, pepper, salt, and broth.
4. Secure the lid and place the pressure valve to seal position.
5. Set to HIGH PRESSURE for 15 min.
6. NPR when the timer beeps; unlock the lid and open.
7. Stir in the cheeses till melted. Add the bacon.
8. Stir to mix.
9. Serve.

Nutrition: Calories 462 - Fats 37 g - Carbs 8 g - Proteins 22 g

176.   SIGNATURE ITALIAN PORK DISH

Prep Time: 15 min   **Cooking Time**: 15 min   **Servings**: 6

Ingredients:

- 2 lb. pork tenderloins, cut into 1½-inch pieces
- ¼ cup almond flour
- 1 tsp. garlic salt
- Freshly ground black pepper, to taste
- 2 tbsp. butter
- ½ cup homemade chicken broth
- ⅓ cup balsamic vinegar
- 1 tbsp. capers
- 2 tsp. fresh lemon zest, grated finely.

Direction:

1. In a large bowl, add the pork pieces, flour, garlic salt, black pepper, and toss to coat well.

2. Remove pork pieces from bowl and shake off excess flour mixture.

3. In a large skillet, melt the butter over medium-high heat and cook the pork pieces for about 2-3 min. per side.

4. Add broth and vinegar and bring to a gentle boil.

5. Reduce the heat to medium and simmer for about 3-4 min.

6. With a slotted spoon, transfer the pork pieces onto a plate.

7. In the same skillet, add the capers, lemon zest, and simmer for about 3-5 min. or until the desired thickness of sauce.

8. Pour sauce over pork pieces and serve.

Nutrition: Calories: 373 kcal Carbs: 1.8 g Fiber: 0.7 g Sugar: 0.4 g Protein: 46.7 g Fat: 18.6 g Sodium: 231 mg.

177. FLAVOR PACKED PORK LOIN

Prep Time: 15 min   **Cooking Time**: 1 h   **Servings**: 6

Ingredients:

- ⅓ cup low-sodium soy sauce
- ¼ cup fresh lemon juice
- 2 tsp. fresh lemon zest, grated
- 1 tbs. fresh thyme, finely chopped
- 2 tbsp. fresh ginger, grated
- 2 garlic cloves, chopped finely
- 2 tbsp. Erythritol
- Freshly ground black pepper, to taste
- ½ tsp. cayenne pepper
- 2 lb. boneless pork loin.

Direction:

1. For pork marinade: in a large baking dish, add all the ingredients except pork loin and mix until well combined. Add the pork loin and coat with the marinade generously.

2. Refrigerate for about 24 hours.

3. Preheat the oven to 400°F.

4. Remove the pork loin from marinade and arrange it into a baking dish.

5. Cover the baking dish and bake for about 1 hour.

6. Remove from the oven and place the pork loin onto a cutting board.

7. With a piece of foil, cover each loin for at least 10 min. before slicing.

8. With a sharp knife, cut the pork loin into desired size slices and serve.

Nutrition: Calories: 230 kcal Carbs: 3.2 g Fiber: 0.6 g Sugar: 1.2 g Protein: 40.8 g Fat: 5.6 g Sodium: 871 mg.

178. SPICED PORK TENDERLOIN

Prep Time: 15 min   **Cooking Time**: 18 min   **Servings**: 6

Ingredients:

- 2 tsp. fresh rosemary, minced
- 2 tsp. fennel seeds
- 2 tsp. coriander seeds
- 2 tsp. caraway seeds
- 1 tsp. cumin seeds
- 1 bay leaf
- Salt and freshly ground black pepper, to taste
- 2 tbsp. fresh dill, chopped
- 1-2 lb. pork tenderloins, trimmed.

Direction:

1. For spice rub: in a spice grinder, add the seeds and bay leaf and grind until finely powdered.

2. Add the salt and black pepper and mix.

3. In a small bowl, reserve 2 tbsp. of spice rub.

4. In another small bowl, mix together the remaining spice rub, and dill.

5. Place 1 tenderloin over a piece of plastic wrap.

6. With a sharp knife, slice through the meat to within ½-inch of the opposite side.

7. Now, open the tenderloin like a book.

8. Cover with another plastic wrap and with a meat pounder, gently pound into ½-inch thickness.

9. Repeat with the remaining tenderloin.

10. Remove the plastic wrap and spread half of the dill mixture over the center of each tenderloin.

11. Roll each tenderloin like a cylinder.

12. With a kitchen string, tightly tie each roll at several places.

13. Rub each roll with the reserved spice rub generously.

14. With 1 plastic wrap, wrap each roll and refrigerate for at least 4-6 hours.

15. Preheat the grill to medium-high heat. Grease the grill grate.

16. Remove the plastic wrap from tenderloins.

17. Place tenderloins onto the grill and cook for about 14-18 min., flipping occasionally.

18. Remove from the grill and place tenderloins onto a cutting board and with a piece of foil, cover each tenderloin for at least 5-10 min. before slicing.

19. With a sharp knife, cut the tenderloins into desired size slices and serve.

Nutrition: Calories: 313 kcal Carbs: 1.4 g Fiber: 0.7 g Sugar: 0 g Protein: 45.7 g Fat: 12.6 g Sodium: 127 mg.

179. STICKY PORK RIBS

Prep Time: 15 min   **Cooking Time:** 2 h 34 min   **Servings:** 9

Ingredients:

- ¼ cup Erythritol
- 1 tbsp. garlic powder
- 1 tbsp. paprika
- ½ tsp. red chili powder
- 4 lb. pork ribs, membrane removed
- Salt and freshly ground black pepper, to taste
- 1½ tsp. liquid smoke
- 1½ cup sugar-free BBQ sauce.

Direction:

1. Preheat the oven to 300°F.

2. Line a large baking sheet with 2 layers of foil, shiny side out. In a bowl, add the Erythritol, garlic powder, paprika, chili powder, and mix well.

3. Season the ribs with salt and black pepper and then, coat with the liquid smoke.

4. Now, rub the ribs with the Erythritol mixture.

5. Arrange the ribs onto the prepared baking sheet, meaty side down.

6. Arrange 2 layers of foil on top of ribs and then, roll and crimp edges tightly.

7. Bake for about 2-2½ hours or until the desired doneness.

8. Remove the baking sheet from oven and place the ribs onto a cutting board.

9. Now, set the oven to broiler.

10. With a sharp knife, cut the ribs into serving sized portions and evenly coat with the barbecue sauce.

11. Arrange the ribs onto a broiler pan, bony side up.

12. Broil for about 1-2 min. per side.

13. Remove from the oven and serve hot.

Nutrition: Calories: 530 kcal Carbs: 2.8 g Fiber: 0.5 g Sugar: 0.4 g Protein: 60.4 g Fat: 40.3 g Sodium: 306 mg.

180. LOW-CALORIE CHEESY BROCCOLI QUICHE

Prep Time: 25 min   **Cooking Time:** 30 min   **Servings:** 2

Ingredients:

- ⅓ tbsp. butter
- Black pepper
- 4 oz. broccoli
- ¼ tsp. garlic powder
- 2 tbsp. full-fat cream
- ⅛ cup scallions
- Kosher salt
- ¼ cup cheddar cheese
- 2 eggs.

Directions:

1. Warm-up, the oven to 360°F, then grease the baking dish with butter.
2. Put broccoli and 4 to 8 tbsp. water and place the bowl in the microwave within 3 min. Mix and again bake within 3 min.
3. Beat the eggs in a bowl. Pour all leftover items with broccoli.
4. Put all mixture in the baking dish. Bake within 30 min. Slice and serve.

Nutrition: Calories: 196 Fats: 14 g Carbs: 5 g Proteins: 12 g Fiber: 2 g.

---

181.   LOW CARB BROCCOLI LEEK SOUP

Prep Time: 15 min   **Cooking Time**: 15 min   **Servings**: 2

Ingredients:

- ½ leek
- 3½ oz. cream cheese
- 5½ oz. broccoli
- ½ cup heavy cream
- 1 cup of water
- ¼ tbsp. black pepper
- ½ vegetable bouillon cube
- ¼ cup basil
- 1 tsp. garlic
- Salt.

Directions:

1. Put water into a pan and put broccoli chopped, leek chopped, and salt.
2. Boil on high.
3. Simmer on low.
4. Put the remaining items, simmer for 1 min. Remove.
5. Blend the soup mixture into a blender. Serve.

Nutrition: Calories: 545 kcal Fats: 50 g Carbs: 10 g Proteins: 15 g.

---

182.   BLACK SOYBEAN SOUP

Prep Time: 10 min.   **Cooking Time**: 40 min.   **Servings**: 4-6

Ingredients:

- 1 small red onion, diced
- 1 tbsp. cumin
- 1/2 tsp. cayenne pepper
- 14 ounces dry black soybeans
- Avocado salsa, for garnish, optional
- 1 red pepper, diced
- 1/2 bunch cilantro leaves & stems, divided
- 2 tbsp. chili powder
- 3 cloves garlic, minced
- 3 cups vegetable broth, plus extra water

Directions:

1. Place the onion, garlic, and cilantro stems in the IP. Add a splash of water.
2. Set the IP to SAUTE; cook for 2 to 3 min. or till translucent. Add the red pepper and spices; sauté for 1 to 2 min.
3. Add the soybeans and broth; stir to mix well.
4. Add enough water to cover the beans with 1-inch water.
5. Secure the lid and place the pressure valve to seal position.
6. Set to MANUAL HIGH PRESSURE for 30 min.
7. QPR when the timer beeps; unlock the lid and open.
8. Puree all or only 1/2 of the soup using an immersion or regular blender.

Nutrition: Calories 174 Fats 7.1 g Carbs 8.6 g Proteins 14.3 g

---

183.   AVOCADO WITH BROCCOLI AND ZUCCHINI SALAD

Prep Time:10 min.   **Cooking Time**: 10 min.   **Servings**: 4

Ingredients:

- 1 large zucchini, julienne
- 1/2 cup broccoli, cut into florets
- 2 avocados, sliced
- 2 cup goat cheese
- 1 tbsp. apple cider vinegar

Directions:

1. Combine zucchini, goat cheese, broccoli, and vinegar, then mix well.
2. Season to taste, and top with avocado slices.
3. Serve, and enjoy.

Nutrition: Calories 215 - Fats 17.6 g - Carbs 6.1 g - Proteins 9.8 g

184.   CREAMY KALE SALAD

Prep Time: 10 min.   **Cooking Time:** 0 min.   **Servings:** 3

Ingredients:

- Kale (2 bunches)
- 1 cup sour cream
- 2 tbsp. sesame seeds oil
- 2 tbsp. lemon juice
- Goat Cheese (6 oz.)

Directions:

1. Chop kale and wash kale then remove the ribs.
2. Transfer kale to a large bowl.
3. Add sour cream, and sesame seeds oil.
4. Season to taste and mix thoroughly.
5. Top with your goat cheese.
6. Serve and enjoy.

Nutrition: Calories 78 - Fats 6.4 g - Carbs 3.2 g - Proteins 1.1 g

185.   CHEESY ROASTED BRUSSELS SPROUT SALAD

Prep Time: 10 min.   **Cooking Time:** 15min.   **Servings:** 2

Ingredients:

- Brussels sprouts (1 lb.)
- 1 tbsp. olive oil
- Feta cheese (1 cup, crumbled)
- Parmesan cheese (¼ cup, grated)
- Hazelnuts (¼ cup, whole, skins removed)

Directions:

1. Set your oven to preheat to 350°F.
2. Line a baking sheet with a silicone baking mat or parchment paper. Trim the bottom and core from each Brussels sprout with a small knife.
3. Put the leaves in a medium bowl; you can use your hands to release all the leaves fully.
4. Toss the leaves with olive oil and season with pink salt and pepper.
5. Add your leaves evenly to the bottom of your baking sheet.
6. Roast for 10 to 15 min., or until lightly browned and crisp.
7. Divide the roasted Brussels sprouts leaves between two bowls, top each with the shaved Parmesan cheese and hazelnuts, and serve.

Nutrition: Calories 287 - Fats 19 g - Carbs 9 g - Proteins 14 g

186.   LETTUCE GROUND BEEF SALAD

Prep Time: 10 min.   **Cooking Time:** 5 min.   **Servings:** 2-3

Ingredients:

- ½ Cup of Grated Cheese
- 2 Cups of Chopped Lettuce
- 1 Medium Avocado
- ½ of a Medium lime
- ½ Cup of Sour Cream
- 2 Tbsp. of chopped Red Onion Chopped
- Sugar-free salsa
- 1 lb. of beef mince
- ¼ tsp of Garlic Powder
- ¼ tsp of dried Oregano
- ½ tsp of Paprika
- 1 and ½ tsp of ground cumin
- ¾ Cup of water

Directions:

1. Heat your Air Fryer to a temperature of about 390°F.
2. Place the meat, the seasoning and 2 tbsp. of water in your Air Fryer Pan.
3. Season the meat with 1 pinch of salt and 1 pinch of ground black pepper.
4. Place the Air Fryer pan in your Air Fryer and lock the lid.
5. Set the timer to about 5 min. and set the temperature to 390°F.
6. When the timer beeps; turn off your Air Fryer.
7. Transfer the ground meat to a serving platter and cover with the chopped lettuce.
8. Season your salad with 1 pinch of salt and drizzle with olive oil.
9. Serve and enjoy your salad!

Nutrition: Calories 310 - Fats 18 g - Carbs 9 g - Proteins 23 g

187. SHRIMP AND AVOCADO LETTUCE CUPS

Prep Time: 10 min. **Cooking Time:** 5 min. **Servings:** 2

Ingredients:

- 1 tbsp. ghee
- ½ pound shrimp
- ½ cup halved grape tomatoes
- ½ avocado, sliced
- 4 butter lettuce leaves, rinsed and patted dry

Directions:

1. In a medium skillet over medium-high heat, heat the ghee. Add the shrimp and cook.
2. Season with pink salt and pepper.
3. Shrimp are cooked when they turn pink and opaque.
4. Season the tomatoes and avocado with pink salt and pepper.
5. Divide the lettuce cups between two plates.
6. Fill each cup with shrimp, tomatoes, and avocado.
7. Drizzle the mayo sauce on top and serve.

Nutrition: Calories 326 - Fats 11 g - Carbs 7 g - Proteins 33 g

188. CLASSIC PORK TENDERLOIN

Prep Time: 15 min **Cooking Time:** 35 min **Servings:** 4

Ingredients:

- 8 bacon slices
- 2 lb. pork tenderloin
- 1 tsp. dried oregano, crushed
- 1 tsp. dried basil, crushed
- 1 tbsp. garlic powder
- 1 tsp. seasoned salt
- 3 tbsp. butter.

Directions:

1. Preheat the oven to 400°F.
2. Heat a large ovenproof skillet over medium-high heat and cook the bacon for about 6-7 min. Transfer the bacon onto a paper towel lined plate to drain.
3. Then, wrap the pork tenderloin with bacon slices and secure with toothpicks. With a sharp knife, slice the tenderloin between each bacon slice to make a medallion.
4. In a bowl, mix together the dried herbs, garlic powder and seasoned salt.

5. Now, coat the medallion with herb mixture.

6. With a paper towel, wipe out the skillet.

7. In the same skillet, melt the butter over medium-high heat and cook the pork medallion for about 4 min. per side.

8. Now, transfer the skillet into the oven.

9. Roast for about 17-20 min.

10. Remove the wok from oven and let it cool slightly before cutting.

11. Cut the tenderloin into desired size slices and serve.

Nutrition: Calories: 471 Fat: 19 g Protein: 9 g Carbs: 8 g Fiber: 3 g.

CHAPTER 12: DESSERTS

189.   MUG CAKE

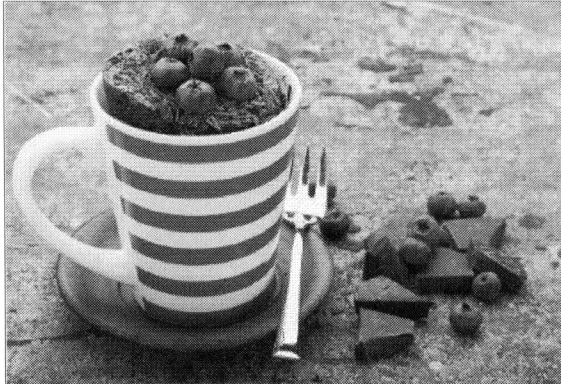

Prep. Time: 5 Min.   **Cooking Time**: 2 Min.   **Servings**: 1

Ingredients:
- 1 egg, lightly beaten
- 1/8 tsp baking powder, gluten-free
- 2 tbsp. creamy peanut butter
- 1 tbsp. Swerve

Directions:
1. Add all ingredients into the microwave-safe mug and stir until well combined.
2. Place mug in microwave and microwave for 1-2 min.
3. Serve and luxuriate in.

Nutrition: Calories 257 - Fats 20.5 g - Carbs 8.9 g - Proteins 13.5 g

190.   CHOCOLATE FAT BOMBS

Prep. Time: 10 Min.   **Cooking Time**: 5 Min   **Servings**: 30

Ingredients:
- 3,5 oz. unsweetened dark chocolate
- 6 drops liquid stevia
- ¼ cup of coconut oil

Directions:
1. Add chocolate, oil, and sweetener in a microwave-safe bowl and microwave until chocolate is melted.
2. Pour chocolate mixture into the mold and place it within the refrigerator until set.
3. Serve and luxuriate in.

Nutrition: Calories 38 - Fats 3.6 g - Carbs 0.9 g - Proteins 0.4 g

191.   DELICIOUS CHOCOLATE FROSTY

Prep. Time: 10 Min.   **Cooking Time**: 10 Min.   **Servings**: 2

Ingredients:
- 1 ½ cups heavy whipping cream
- 2 ½ tbsp. monk fruit
- 1 tbsp. vanilla
- 2 tbsp. unsweetened cocoa powder

Directions:
1. Add all ingredients into the massive bowl.
2. Beat using the hand mixer until peaks form.
3. Scoop the mixture into the zip-lock bag and place it within the refrigerator for 45 min.
4. Remove a zip-lock bag from the refrigerator and cut the corner of the pack.
5. Squeeze frosty in serving bowls.
6. Serve chilled.

Nutrition: Calories 342 - Fats 34 g - Carbs 6.3 g - Proteins 2.9 g

192.   STRAWBERRY MOUSSE

Prep. Time: 10 Min.   **Cooking Time**: 5 Min.   **Servings**: 4

Ingredients:
- 1 cup heavy whipping cream
- 1 cup fresh strawberries, chopped
- 2 tbsp. Swerve
- 1 cup cream cheese

Directions:
1.   Add heavy light whipping cream during a large bowl and beat until thickened using a hand mixer.

2. Add sweetener and cheese and beat well.
3. Add strawberries and fold well.
4. Pour in serving glasses and place them within the refrigerator for 1-2 hours.
5. Serve chilled and luxuriate in.

Nutrition: Calories 320 - Fats 31.4 g - Carbs 6.2 g - Proteins 5.2 g

193. CHEESECAKE MOUSSE

Prep. Time: 10 Min. **Cooking Time**: 5 Min. **Servings**: 6

Ingredients:

- 1 cup heavy whipping cream
- 1 tsp vanilla
- ¼ cup erythritol
- 8 oz. cream cheese, softened

Directions:

1. Add the cheese to a bowl and beat until smooth. Add vanilla and sweetener and stir to mix.
2. In another bowl, beat heavy light whipping cream until stiff peaks form.
3. Fold topping into the cheese mixture and beat employing a hand mixer until fluffy.
4. Place in the refrigerator for two hours.
5. Pipe in serving glasses and serve chilled.

Nutrition: Calories 203 - Fats 20.6 g - Carbs 11.7 g - Proteins 3.3 g

194. BERRY CHEESE DESSERT

Prep. Time: 10 Min. **Cooking Time**: 10 Min. **Servings**: 8

Ingredients:

- 1 ½ lb. ricotta cheese
- 1 cup blackberries
- 1 cup blueberries
- 1 cup raspberries
- 1 ½ tsp vanilla
- ½ cup erythritol
- 1 tbsp. lemon zest
- ¼ cup heavy cream

Directions:

1. Add ricotta, vanilla, sweetener, and cream in a bowl and using a hand mixer, beat until smooth.
2. In four serving cups, place in layer alternating the ricotta mixture and ¼ cup of berries.
3. Serve and luxuriate in.

Nutrition: Calories 201 - Fats 12 g - Carbs 9 g - Proteins 10 g

195. PANCAKES WITH WHIPPED CREAM AND BERRIES

Prep Time: 5 Min. **Cooking Time**: 20 Min. **Servings** 4

Ingredients:

- 4 eggs, beaten
- 7 ounces (198 g) cottage cheese
- 1 tbsp. ground psyllium husk powder
- 2 ounces (57 g) butter or coconut oil
- 1 cup heavy whipping cream
- 2 ounces (57 g) fresh raspberries or blueberries

Directions:

1. Mix all the ingredients except the butter together in a bowl and let it rest for 5 to 10 min. to thicken.
2. Put the butter or coconut oil on a nonstick skillet. Scoop some of the batter on the skillet and let it fry for 3 to 4 min. on each side over medium-low heat. Don't let it be too big to make it easy to flip.
3. Pour some cream into a separate bowl and whisk until soft peaks are formed.
4. Serve the pancakes with the whipped cream and some berries on the side.

Nutrition: Calories: 413 Fat: 37 Fiber: 3g Net Carbs: 2g Protein: 15.3g

196.   CHEESY SHELLS
Prep Time: 40 Min.   **Cooking Time**: 20 Min.   **Servings** 12
Ingredients:

- 3 ounces (85 g) cream cheese, softened
- ½ cup butter, softened
- ¼ cup coconut flour

SPECIAL EQUIPMENT: - Mini muffin cups

Directions:
1. Preheat the oven to 325°F (160°C).
2. Mix the cream cheese with the butter in a bowl until well combined then add the flour. Mix until well blended then put it in the refrigerator to chill for 1 hour.
3. Roll the chilled dough into 24 1-inch (2.5 cm) balls then press each ball into each ungreased mini muffin cups to make a shallow shell. Fill the shell with your desired fillings and bake it for 20 min. or until the crust is light brown.
4. Serve with your favorite toppings.
5. To make this a complete meal, serve it with a creamy topping and some berries

Nutrition: Calories: 90 Fat: 9.7g Carbs: 0.4 Protein 0.6g Cholesterol: 27mg Sodium: 97mg

197.   CHEWY NUTTY CHOCOLATE CUBES
Prep Time: 10 Min.   **Cooking Time**: 35 Min.   **Servings** 12
Ingredients:

- ounces (99 g) dark chocolate with a minimum of 80% cocoa solids
- 4 tbsp. butter or coconut oil
- ¼ cup peanut butter
- 1 pinch salt
- ½ tsp. vanilla extract
- 1 tsp. licorice powder or ground cinnamon or ground cardamom (green)
- 1.5 ounces (43 g) hazelnuts, finely chopped

Directions:
1. Put the chocolate and butter or coconut oil in a microwave-safe bowl and put it in the microwave to melt. Stir well to make sure it is combined then, set aside.
2. Mix in the rest of the ingredients except the hazelnuts until well blended.
3. Grease a dish and line with parchment paper then pour the batter into the dish.
4. Sprinkle the chopped hazelnuts over the batter then place it in the refrigerator to chill.
5. When it has hardened, cut it into cubes and store it in the refrigerator or freezer. Serve cold.

Nutrition: Calories: 139 Fat: 11g Fiber: 2g Net Carbs: 3g Protein: 4g

198.   CREAMY CHOCOLATE CAKE
Prep Time: 5 Min.   **Cooking Time**: 15 Min.   **Servings** 12
Ingredients:

- 7 ounces (198 g) sugar-free dark chocolate| stevia sweetened
- 7 ounces (198 g) hazelnuts
- ounces (99 g) pumpkin seeds
- 3 tbsp. erythritol
- 1¼ cups heavy whipping cream or coconut cream
- 7 tbsp. butter
- 1 pinch sea salt

SPECIAL EQUIPMENT: - A spring-form pan

Directions:
1. Pour the heavy cream and the erythritol into a saucepan then bring to a boil on low heat for 3 to 5 min. until it is creamy and turn off the heat.
2. Chop the chocolate and the butter into smaller pieces and add it to the cream. Mix in the salt until everything is well combined.
3. Pour the hazelnuts and pumpkin seeds on a large frying pan and let it roast until it is

golden and fragrant. Roughly chop them with a knife then add it to the chocolate mix. Reserve some chopped hazelnuts and pumpkin seeds for topping.

4. Cover a spring-form pan with parchment paper and spoon the mixture on the pan then

sprinkle the top with the roasted nuts and seeds you have reserved.

5. Cover the pan with a thin film and put in the fridge for 1 hour or until thoroughly hardened.

6. Serve cold.

Nutrition: Calories: 410 Fat: 38g Fiber: 4g Net Carbs: 5g Protein: 9g

---

199. VANILLA CHEESECAKES

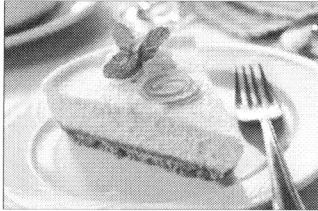

Prep Time: 10 Min.   **Cooking Time**: 15 Min.   **Servings** 12

Ingredients:

- ½ cup almond meal
- ¾ tsp. liquid stevia
- 1 tsp. vanilla extract
- ¼ cup butter, melted
- 2 (8 ounces / 227 g) packages cream cheese| softened
- 2 eggs
- 12 Muffin cups

SPECIAL EQUIPMENT

Directions:

1. Preheat the oven to 350°F (180°C) and line 12 muffin cups with paper liners.
2. Combine the almond meal and the butter in a bowl then scoop the mixture into the bottom of each muffin cup and press until it is a flat crust. Whisk the cream cheese, eggs, stevia, and vanilla extract together in a separate bowl until it is smooth with a mixer. Scoop the mixture into each of the muffin cups.
3. Bake in the oven for 15 to 17 min. then dip a toothpick into the middle to check the doneness. It should come out clean.
4. Let it cool then refrigerate for at least 8 hours before serving.

SERVE IT WITH: To make this a complete meal, serve it with a dollop of sour cream.

Nutrition: Calories: 221 Fat: 21g Carbs: 3.3g Protein: 4.7g Cholesterol: 81mg Sodium: 152mg

---

200. CHOCOLATE PEANUT BUTTER FUDGE

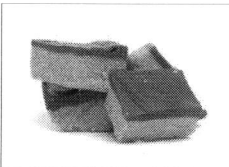

Prep. Time: 10 Min.   **Cooking Time**: 10 Min.   **Servings**: 16

Ingredients:

- ½ cup peanut butter
- ½ tsp vanilla
- ¼ cup Swerve
- 2 ½ tbsp. unsweetened cocoa powder
- ¼ cup ghee

Directions:

1. Line a small baking dish with parchment paper and put it aside.
2. Add ghee a spread in a microwave-safe bowl and microwave until ghee and spread are melted.
3. Add remaining ingredients and stir everything well and pour in a prepared baking dish.
4. Place in refrigerator for 1 hour or until set.
5. Dig pieces and serve.

Nutrition: Calories 78 - Fats 7.4 g - Carbs 2.1 g - Proteins 2.2 g

---

201. RASPBERRY FAT BOMBS

Prep. Time: 5 Min.   **Cooking Time**: 5 Min.   **Servings**: 8

Ingredients:

- ½ cup fresh raspberries
- 3 tbsp. Swerve
- 2 tbsp. coconut oil, melted
- 8 oz. cream cheese, softened

Directions:

1. Add all ingredients into the kitchen appliance and process until smooth.
2. Pour the fat bomb mixture into the mini muffin mold and place it within the refrigerator for 45 min.
3. Serve and luxuriate in.

Nutrition: Calories 134 - Fats 13.3 g - Carbs 2.4 g - Proteins 2.2 g

202.   QUICK LEMON MUG CAKE

Prep. Time: 5 Min.   **Cooking Time**: 2 Min.   **Servings**: 1

Ingredients:

- 1 egg, lightly beaten
- ½ tsp lemon rind
- 1 tbsp. butter, melted
- 1 ½ tbsp. fresh lemon juice
- 2 tbsp. erythritol
- ¼ tsp baking powder, gluten-free
- ¼ cup almond flour

Directions:

1. During a small bowl, mix almond flour, leaven, and sweetener.
2. Add egg, juice, and melted butter in almond flour mixture and whisk until well combined.
3. Pour cake mixture into the microwave-safe mug and microwave for 90 seconds.
4. Serve and luxuriate in.

Nutrition: Calories 385 - Fats 32 g - Carbs 8 g - Proteins 13 g

203.   SMOOTH & SILKY TIRAMISU MOUSSE

Prep. Time: 5 Min.   **Cooking Time**: 5 Min.   **Servings**: 2

Ingredients:

- ½ cup mascarpone cheese
- 1 tbsp. erythritol
- 1 tsp unsweetened cocoa powder

Directions:

1. Add all ingredients into the blender and blend until smooth. Pour blended mixture into the piping bag and pipe in serving glasses.
2. Place in refrigerator for 1 hour.
3. Serve chilled and luxuriate in.

Nutrition: Calories 110 - Fats 8.2 g - Carbs 2.4 g - Proteins 7.2 g

204.   ALMOND MUG CAKE

Prep. Time: 8-10 Min.   **Cooking Time**: 10 Min.   **Servings**: 1

Ingredients:

- 1/4 tsp. baking powder
- 1/4 tsp. vanilla extract
- 1 1/2 tbsp. cacao powder
- 1 egg, beaten
- 1/4 cup almond flour
- 1 tsp. cinnamon powder
- 2 tbsp. stevia powder
- A pinch of salt

Directions:

1. Combine all ingredients within the bowl until well-combined. Add the combination during a heat-proof mug, cover with a foil.
2. Arrange Instant Pot over a dry platform in your kitchen. Open its top lid and switch it on.
3. Within the pot, pour water. Arrange a trivet or steamer basket inside that came with Instant Pot. Now place/arrange the mug over the trivet/basket.
4. Close the lid to make a locked chamber; confirm that the relief valve is in a locking position.
5. Find and press "MANUAL" cooking function; timer to 10 min. with default "HIGH" pressure mode.
6. Allow the pressure to create to cook the ingredients.
7. After cooking time is over, press the "CANCEL" setting. Find and press the "QPR" cooking function.

8. This setting is for the quick release of inside pressure.

9. Slowly open the lid, calm down the mug, and serve warm.

Nutrition: Calories 138 - Fats 13 g - Carbs 7 g - Fiber 3 g - Proteins 9 g

205. CREAMY VANILLA CHOCOLATE BOWLS

Prep. Time: 15 Min.   **Cooking Time**: 20 Min.   **Servings** 16

Ingredients:

DARK CHOCOLATE CAKE:

- 9 ounces (255 g) dark chocolate with a minimum of 70% cocoa solids
- 5 ounces (142 g) butter
- 5 eggs
- 1 pinch salt
- 1 tsp. vanilla extract

FOR SERVINGS:

- 8 ounces (227 g) fresh raspberries or fresh blueberries
- 6 tbsp. lime juice
- 1 tsp. vanilla extract
- 2 cups heavy whipping cream
- 4 ounces (113 g) pecans, chopped
- 1.5 ounces (43 g) roasted unsweetened coconut chips

SPECIAL EQUIPMENT:

- A spring form pan

Directions:

1. Heat the oven to 325°F(160°C).
2. Grease a spring form pan with butter or coconut oil then line it with parchment paper.
3. Cut the chocolate and the butter into smaller pieces and melt it together in a heat-safe bowl in the microwave. Set aside to cool.
4. Break the eggs and remove the yolks from the egg whites and put them in separate bowls.

Sprinkle some salt in the egg whites then whisk until soft peaks form and keep aside.

5. Pour the vanilla extract into the yolks and whisk well.
6. Add the chocolate mixture to the yolks and mix well then fold in the egg whites. Pour the mixture into the pan and bake for 15 to 20 min. or until a toothpick inserted into the cake comes out clean.

TO SERVE:

1. Combine the berries, lime juice and vanilla in a small bowl then set aside for 5 min.
2. Whisk the cream in a large bowl until soft peaks are formed.
3. Cut the chocolate cake into small bite sizes and share into plates.
4. Put some berries and sprinkle some coconut flakes over it. Serve immediately.

TIPS: To make this a complete meal, serve immediately with a generous amount of whipped cream.

Nutrition: Calories: 356 Fat: 32g Net Carbs: 8g Protein: 6g Fiber: 2g

206. MACADAMIA CHOCO BOMBS

Prep Time: 10 Min.   **Cooking Time**: 30 Min.   **Servings** 4

Ingredients:

- 1.5 ounces (43 g) raw macadamia nut halves
- 1.3 ounces (37 g) sugar-free dark chocolate, or stevia-sweetened chocolate chips
- 1 tbsp. MCT oil or coconut oil
- Coarse salt or sea salt, to taste

SPECIAL EQUIPMENT:

- Truffle mold, mini muffin pan, or mini baking cups that have 2" × 1" (5 × 2.5 cm) wells

Directions:

1. Put 3 raw macadamia nut halves in 8 of the cups or the mold.
2. Pour the chocolate chips in a microwave-safe bowl and microwave it for 50 seconds or until

it has melted. Stir until it is smooth then add the coconut oil and a pinch of salt. Mix well.

3. Divide and scoop some of the mixture into

each mold making sure the chocolate covers the nuts completely.

4. Put the mold or cups in the freezer to freeze for 30 min. or until it is solid.

5. Remove them from the freezer and serve cold.

Nutrition: Calories: 167 Fat: 15g Fiber: 3g Net Carbs: 2g Protein: 1g

---

207. KETO CHOCOLATE MUG MUFFINS

Prep Time: 5 Min.   **Cooking Time:** 2 Min.   **Servings** 4

Ingredients:

- 4 tbsp. almond flour or hazelnut flour
- 2 tbsp. cocoa powder
- 4 tbsp. erythritol
- 1 tsp. baking powder
- ½ tsp. vanilla extract
- 2 pinches salt
- 2 eggs, beaten
- 3 tbsp. melted coconut oil or butter
- 1 tsp. coconut oil or butter, for greasing the mugs
- 0.5 ounce (14 g) sugar-free dark chocolate, chopped

SPECIAL EQUIPMENT:

- 4 greased coffee mugs or ramekins, or a 4-cup muffin tin

Directions:

TO COOK IN A MICROWAVE:

1. In a small bowl, mix the flour, cocoa powder, erythritol, baking powder, vanilla extract, and salt. Mix in the eggs, butter, and chocolate until the batter is smooth then set aside.

2. Pour the batter equally into four greased coffee mugs or ramekins.
3. Put them in the microwave and cook for 1.5 min. at high pressure. Remove the mugs and let it cool for 1min. Serve warm.

TO BAKE IN AN OVEN:

1. Preheat the oven to 350°F (180°C).
2. Mix the flour, cocoa powder, erythritol, baking powder, vanilla extract, and salt in a small bowl and add the eggs, oil or butter and chocolate. Mix it until it is smooth and set aside.

3. Line a 4-cup muffin tin with liners and pour the batter into the tin until it is filled halfway.
4. Bake for 12 to 14 min. or until it is springy in the middle and an inserted toothpick comes out clean. Remove from the oven and serve warm.

TIPS: To make this a complete meal, serve it with a generous amount of heavy whipped cream.

Nutrition: Calories: 208 Fat: 18g Fiber: 2g Net Carbs: 1g Protein: 4g

---

208. LEMONY BLUEBERRY ICE CREAM

Prep Time: 50 Min.   **Cooking Time:** 0 Min.   **Servings** 14

Ingredients:

- 2 cups blueberries
- 2 tbsp. roasted and finely ground flax seeds
- 2 (15 ounces / 425 g) cans coconut milk, chilled
- 1 tbsp. lemon juice
- 1 tsp. vanilla extract
- 1 tsp. coconut oil
- 1 tsp. stevia powder
- ½ tsp. xanthan gum, or more as desired
- ¼ tsp. Himalayan black salt

Directions:

1. Put the flax seeds in a coffee grinder and pulse till it is smooth.
2. Mix one can of coconut milk with blueberries, and lemon juice in a blender and puree till the

blueberry skins break down completely. Add the ground flax seeds, rest of the coconut milk, vanilla, oil, stevia powder, xanthan gum, and salt to the blender and puree until smooth.

3. Pour the mixture into a pan and put it in the freezer to chill for 15 min.

4. Pour it into an ice cream maker and churn for 20 min.

5. Remove the ice cream from the machine into a lidded container and serve

Nutrition: Calories: 141 Fat: 12.8g Carbs: 4.5g Protein: 1.5g Cholesterol: 0mg Sodium: 50mg

---

209. CINNAMON AND PECAN BARS

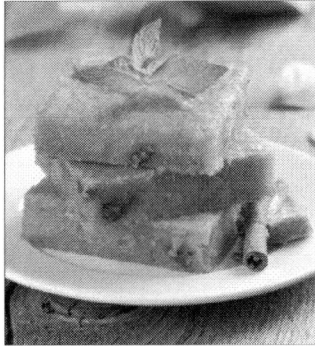

Prep Time: 15 Min.   **Cooking Time**: 35 Min.   **Servings** 16

Ingredients:

- 1 cup pecans
- 1 tsp.
- 1 tsp. ground cinnamon
- ¼ tsp. ground nutmeg
- 2 tbsp. melted butter
- 4 eggs
- ¼ cup cream cheese
- ¼ cup sour cream
- ¼ tsp. vanilla extract
- 1 cup unsweetened almond milk

liquid stevia

SYRUP:

- 1 cup fresh strawberries
- 1 tsp. vanilla
- 2 tbsp. erythritol

SPECIAL EQUIPMENT:
- Brownie pan

Directions:

1. Preheat the oven to 350°F (180°C).
2. Put the pecans in a food processor and blend until it is smooth. Pour in the stevia, cinnamon, and nutmeg then process for 15 seconds. Pour the mixture into a bowl then mix in the melted butter. Pour it into a brownie pan with the divider removed then press it so that it sits in the bottom of the pan.
3. In a separate bowl, beat the eggs with a mixer until it is fluffy then add the cream cheese in small quantities, until the cream cheese is smooth. Mix in the sour cream, vanilla extract, and almond milk until it is smooth. Pour it over the crust in the pan and place the divider into the pan.
4. Put the pan in the oven to bake for 35 min. or until an inserted toothpick comes out clean.
5. Make the syrup: Place a pot over medium heat and add strawberries, vanilla, and erythritol to the pot to cook for 5 min. Stir and crush some of the berries until syrup is formed. Cook until it thickens for 10 min.
6. Remove the cheesecake bars and set aside to cool for 1 hour. Pour the syrup over the bars and slice to serve.

Nutrition: Calories: 120 Fat: 10.3g Carbs: 3.1g Protein: 3.8g Cholesterol 165mg Sodium 63mg

---

210. STRAWBERRY SAUCE

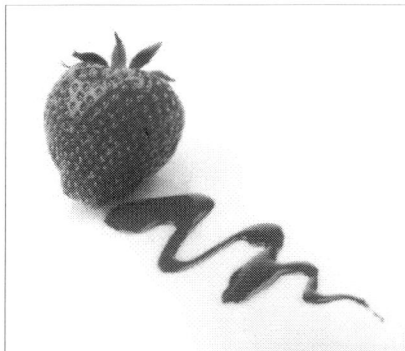

Prep Time: 15 Min.   **Cooking Time**: 20 Min.   **Servings** 4

Ingredients:

- 1 pint fresh strawberries
- 1 tsp. vanilla
- ⅓ cup liquid stevia

Directions:

1. Remove the stems of the strawberries and wash them well then cut them in half or chop them roughly.
2. Mix the strawberries, vanilla, and stevia in a saucepan over medium-high heat. Stir occasionally. It will sizzle for a while and begin to juice. Continue stirring and mash the berries with a spatula to get syrup. Continue to cook for 15 min. or until the sauce thickens.
3. Remove and pour ⅓ of the sauce in a blender. Puree it then pour it unto the rest of the sauce. Store in a fridge.
4. To make this a complete meal, serve it with pies or ice cream.

Nutrition: Calories: 77 Fat: 5g Carbs: 8.1g Protein: 1.1g Cholesterol: 0mg Sodium: 1mg

211.   TAPIOCA KETO PUDDING

Prep Time: 8-10 min.   **Cooking Time**: 20 min.   **Servings**: 4

Ingredients:

- 1 tbsp. Erythritol
- 1 tsp. chia seeds
- 1 tbsp. tapioca
- 1 tbsp. butter
- 2 cup heavy cream
- 1/4 cup raspberries or strawberries, mashed

Directions:

1. Arrange Instant Pot over a dry platform in your kitchen. Open its top lid and switch it on.
2. Find and press the "SAUTE" cooking function. Within the pot, add the cream; cook (while stirring) for 4-5 min.
3. Add the tapioca and stir it well. Add the Erythritol and butter.
4. In a bowl, mix the chia seeds and berries.
5. Add the berry mix within the pot and stir well.
6. Close the lid to make a locked chamber; confirm that the relief valve is in a locking position.
7. Find and press "MANUAL" cooking function; timer to fifteen min.with default "HIGH" pressure mode.
8. Allow the pressure to create to cook the ingredients.
9. After cooking time is over, press the "CANCEL" setting. Find and press the "QPR" cooking function. This setting is for the quick release of inside pressure.
10. Add in serving bowls, calm down, and place within the fridge for two hours.
11. Serve chilled.

Nutrition: Calories 246 - Fats 24 g - Carbs 10 g - Fiber 2 g - Proteins 3 g

212.   CREAM CHOCOLATE DELIGHT

Prep Time: 8-10 min.   **Cooking Time**: 15 min.   **Servings**: 4

Ingredients:

- 1 tsp. orange zest
- 1 tsp. stevia powder
- 2 heavy cream
- ¼ cup unsweetened dark chocolate, chopped
- 3 eggs
- 1 tsp. vanilla extract
- ½ tsp. salt

Directions:

1. Arrange Instant Pot over a dry platform in your kitchen. Open its top lid and switch it on.
2. Find and press the "SAUTE" cooking function.
3. Within the pot, add the cream, chopped chocolate, stevia powder, vanilla, orange peel, and salt; cook (while stirring) until the chocolate is melted.
4. Crack eggs within the pot, stirring constantly. Remove from the moment pot. Add the mixture to 4 mason jars with loose lids.
5. Within the pot, pour water. Arrange a trivet or steamer basket inside that came with Instant Pot. Now place/arrange the jars over the trivet/basket.
6. Close the lid to make a locked chamber; confirm that the relief valve is in a locking position.
7. Find and press "MANUAL" cooking function; timer to 10 min.with default "HIGH" pressure mode.
8. Allow the pressure to create to cook the ingredients.
9. After cooking time is over, press the "CANCEL" setting. Find and press the "QPR" cooking function. This setting is for the quick release of inside pressure.
10. Slowly open the lid, calm down the jars, and chill within the fridge. Serve chilled.

Nutrition: Calories 254 Fats 26 g Carbs 5 g Fiber 1 g Proteins 8 g

213.   COCONUT KETO PUDDING

Prep Time: 8-10 min.   **Cooking Time**: 5 min.   **Servings**: 4

Ingredients:

- 3 tbsp. Stevia granular
- 1/2 tsp. vanilla extract
- 1 2/3 cup coconut milk
- 3 egg yolks
- 1 tbsp. gelatin

Directions:

1. Arrange Instant Pot over a dry platform in your kitchen. Open its top lid and switch it on.
2. Add the coconut milk. Close the lid to make a locked chamber; confirm that the relief valve is in a locking position.
3. Find and press "MANUAL" cooking function; timer to five min.with default "HIGH" pressure mode.
4. Allow the pressure to create to cook the ingredients.
5. After cooking time is over, press the "CANCEL" setting. Find and press the "QPR" cooking function. This setting is for the quick release of inside pressure. Place the coconut milk within the Instant Pot. Close the lid and confirm that the steam release valve is about to "Sealing."
6. Whisk in egg yolks and, therefore, the remainder of the ingredients.
7. Find and press the "SAUTE" cooking function. Cook until boiling the combination.
8. Add in serving bowls, calm down, and place within the fridge for two hours.
9. Serve chilled.

Nutrition: Calories 246 - Fats 27 g - Carbs 7 g - Fiber 4 g - Proteins 4 g

214. CHOCOLATE CAKE

Prep Time: 3 min. **Cooking Time**: 10 min. **Servings**: 4

Ingredients:

- ½ cup raw unsweetened cocoa powder
- ¼ cup butter, melted
- 4 eggs
- ¼ cup sugar-free and gluten-free chocolate sauce
- ½ tsp. ground cinnamon
- ½ tsp. of sea salt
- 1 tsp. pure vanilla extract
- ¼ cup raw stevia

Directions:

1. Pour 1 tbsp. of chocolate sauce into 4 cavities of an ice cube tray and freeze it. Preheat oven to 350°F. Prepare 4 ramekins by greasing with oil or butter.
2. Whisk together the cocoa powder, stevia, cinnamon, and sea salt in a small bowl. Whisk in the eggs, one at a time. Add the melted butter and vanilla extract. Stir until well combined.
3. Fill each prepared ramekin halfway with the mixture.
4. Remove the chocolate sauce from the freezer and place one in each of the ramekins.
5. Cover the chocolate with the remaining cake batter.
6. Bake for 13 to 14 min. or until just set. Transfer from the oven to a wire rack and allow to cool for 5 min.
7. Carefully remove the cakes from the ramekins.
8. Enjoy your tasty and healthy chocolate lava cake by cutting into its molten center.

Nutrition: Calories 189 - Fats 17 g - Carbs 6 g - Fiber 3 g - Proteins 8 g

215. CHOCOLATE CREAM CAKE

Prep Time: 30 min. **Cooking Time**: 30 min. **Servings**: 8

Ingredients:

- 4 ounces unsweetened chocolate
- ½ cup (1 stick) butter
- 1 ½ cups powdered sweetener, divided
- 3 eggs
- ½ cup + 8 tbsp. raw unsweetened cocoa powder
- 1 vanilla pod
- Pinch of sea salt
- 1 cup whipping cream
- Coconut whipped cream
- 1 can coconut milk, refrigerated overnight

Directions:

1. Preheat the oven to 325°F. Spray a little cooking oil into a pan smaller than 8 inches.

2. Combine the chocolate and butter in a double boiler and melt them together. Stir in ½ cup of sweetener and keep on stirring over low heat until everything is well combined. Remove from heat and let cool a little bit.
3. Separate the eggs, and beat the whites until stiff peaks form. Add ¼ cup of sweetener little by little.
4. Whisk the yolks together with another ¼ cup of sweetener. Add the chocolate mixture to the yolks and stir well. Mix in ½ cup cocoa, and then scrape the vanilla seeds from the pod and add to the mix and salt.
5. Fold in egg whites slowly to the chocolate mixture, but do not over mix.
6. Cook in the preheated oven for 1 hour or until a toothpick comes out clean. Let it cool completely and then remove it from the pan.

Cream:
1. To prepare the 3 types of filling, beat the whipping cream for about 6-7 min. until it gets very thick. Slowly add ½ cup of sweetener.
2. Divide the cream into halves and place one half in a bowl. Divide the remaining cream into halves again and place it in the other 2 separate bowls. You will have 3 bowls, one with ½ of the cream and two with ¼ of the cream.
3. Take a bowl with ¼ cream, add 1 tbsp. of cocoa powder and mix well. This will be the lightest-colored cream.
4. Add ½ the cream to the bowl, add 3 tbsp. of cocoa powder. Mix until well distributed. This will be the middle-colored cream.
5. Add 3–4 tbsp. of cocoa powder to the last bowl with ¼ cream. This will be the darkest cream.

Assembling:
1. Slice the cake horizontally in 3 equal slices using a very sharp knife.
2. Place the bottom part on a serving plate and cover with the middle-colored cream. Repeat with the second layer.
3. Top with the third cake piece and spread the light-colored cream on top, followed by the darkest cream.
4. Cut in 8 slices and enjoy.

Nutrition: Calories 304 Fats 27 g Carbs 11 g Fiber 6 g Proteins 7g

216. STRAWBERRY CHEESECAKES

Prep Time: 10 min.   **Cooking Time:** 0 min.   **Servings:** 4

Ingredients:

Crust
- ½ cup almond flour
- 3 tbsp. butter, melted (use coconut oil for a paleo version)
- ¼ cup sugar substitute (use pure Grade B maple syrup for a paleo version)

Filling
- 6 strawberries
- 3 tbsp. sugar substitute (use pure Grade B maple syrup for a paleo version)
- 8 ounces cream cheese (use full-fat unsweetened coconut cream for a paleo version)
- 1/3 cup sour cream (eliminate for a paleo version)
- ½ tsp. pure vanilla extract
- 4 strawberries, quartered (for garnish)
- Fresh mint leaves (optional for garnish)

Directions:
1. To prepare the crust, place the almond flour, melted butter, and sugar substitute in a medium bowl and mix well to combine.
2. Divide the mixture evenly into 4 small serving bowls or ramekins, lightly pressing with your hands.
3. To prepare the filling, puree the strawberries in a food processor.
4. Add the sugar substitute, vanilla extract, cream cheese, and sour cream. Blend until smooth and creamy. Spoon the mixture over the crust and chill for at least 1 hour.

Nutrition: Calories 489 - Fats 47 g - Carbs 12 g - Fiber 3 g - Proteins 8 g

217. BROWNIE CHEESECAKE BARS

Prep Time: 5 min.   **Cooking Time:** 50 min.   **Servings:** 6

Ingredients:

Brownie layer:
- 2 ounces bittersweet chocolate, chopped
- ½ cup butter softened
- ⅓ cup raw unsweetened cocoa powder
- ½ cup almond flour
- 2 large eggs
- ½ cup sugar substitute
- ½ tsp. pure vanilla extract

- ¼ tsp. salt

Cheesecake layer
- 2 large eggs
- 16 ounces cream cheese, softened
- ⅓ cup sugar substitute
- ¼ cup heavy cream
- ½ tsp. pure vanilla extract

Directions:

1. Preheat oven to 325°F.
2. Grease an 8x8 glass baking dish with butter or oil.
3. Melt the chocolate and butter together in a small saucepan over medium heat.
4. Stir until well combined.
5. Whisk the almond flour, cocoa powder, and salt together in a small bowl.
6. Whisk the eggs, sugar substitute, and vanilla extract in a large bowl until frothy.
7. Slowly whisk in the melted chocolate mixture.
8. Stir in the almond flour mixture and mix until smooth.
9. Pour into the prepared baking dish and bake for 20 min. Transfer to a wire rack and allow to cool.
10. For the cheesecake layer, mix the cream cheese, eggs, sugar substitute, heavy cream, and vanilla extract with an electric mixer.
11. Reduce the oven heat to 300°F.
12. Pour the batter over the baked brownies and return to the oven for 40 to 45 min. or until set.
13. Remove from the oven and cool in the fridge for at least 2 hours before serving.

Nutrition: Calories 566- Fats 54 g - Carbs 12 g - Fiber 3 g - Proteins 13 g

218. CHOCOLATE PUDDING

Prep Time: 5 min. **Cooking Time:** 5 min. **Servings:** 4

Ingredients:

- 2 cups coconut milk, canned
- ¼ cup raw unsweetened cocoa powder
- 1 tbsp. stevia
- 2 tbsp. gelatin
- 4 tbsp. water
- ½ cup heavy whipping cream, beaten to stiff peaks
- 1 ounce chopped bittersweet chocolate (optional for garnish)

Directions:

1. Heat the coconut milk, cocoa powder, and stevia in a small saucepan over medium heat.
2. Stir until the cocoa powder and stevia have dissolved.
3. Mix the gelatin with the water and add to the saucepan.
4. Stir until well combined.
5. Pour the mixture into 4 small ramekins or glasses.
6. Place the ramekins in the refrigerator for at least 1 hour.
7. Top with whipped cream, and chopped chocolate, if desired.

Nutrition: Calories 389 -Fats 37 g Carbs 14 g Fiber 5 g Proteins 8 g

219. STRAWBERRIES WITH COCONUT WHIP

Prep Time: 5 min. **Cooking Time:** 3 min. **Servings:** 4

Ingredients:

- 2 cans coconut cream, refrigerated
- 4 cups strawberries (can also use blueberries, blackberries, raspberries, or a combination)
- 1 ounce chopped unsweetened 70% or darker dark chocolate

Directions:

1. Scoop the solidified coconut cream (reserving the liquid in the bottom of the can for another use) into a large bowl and blend with a hand mixer on high for about 5 min. or until stiff peaks form.
2. Slice the strawberries and arrange them in 4 small serving bowls.
3. Dollop the coconut whipped cream on top of the strawberries.
4. Garnish with chopped dark chocolate and additional berries.
5. Serve and enjoy!

Nutrition: Calories 342 - Fats 31 g - Carbs 15 g - Fiber 5 g - Proteins 4 g

CHAPTER 13: 28-DAYS MEAL PLAN

WEEK 1

DAY 1

BREAKFAST

220.   KETO COFFEE

Prep. Time: 45 seconds
Cooking time: 60seconds
Servings: 2

Ingredient:
- 2 tbsp. organic coconut oil (or MCT oil)
- 1 tsp. vanilla extract (optional)
- 2 cups of coffee
- 2 tbsp. grass-fed of unsalted butter
- 1 tbsp. heavy whipping cream (Optional)

Direction:
1. Brew 2 cups of coffee with your preferred form into a big container. Try to pick something big enough (like a measuring jug) to prevent spill when we mix it.
2. If you use a pour-over process, my suggestion is the size of kosher (or somewhat smaller) salt to grind. Fill your coffee filter and wet the coffee with a little water and let it "bloom" for about 30 seconds. Then brew normally in a circular movement by pouring the sugar, carefully ensuring the coffee does not swim in sugar. Take your butter, cocoon oil and dip blender. If you like, you can mix it in a standard blender, but I feel it's more troublemaking than cleaning in a normal blender.
3. Cut 2 tbsp. Cut off of butter fed with hay. I'm shocked how few people use markings for packages – they just cut it in, they work! I like salted butter personally, but many do not. Feel free to start checking unsalted first.
4. Low the butter and add 1 tsp. Vanilla extract and 2 tbsp plunk. Coconut oil (or MCT oil if you need it) too. Finally, but not least, the 1 Tbsp. Strong cream. Heavy cream. This makes the coffee so smooth for a silky feel.
5. Mix it all with your immersion mixer. Usually, the top gets a large frothy cap between 45-60 seconds. Make sure the immersion blender is rotated up and down to emulsify all the fat in the coffee. This would also ventilate the mixture by adding extra froth. Note: You can do it all with a regular blender bottle and mixer ball, so you don't have to shake fats every few min.
6. Look out for the froth (it may drop down the side), but your keto proof coffee is done! Measure it and drink it in your favorite tub.

Nutrition: Calories260 Fats27.7g Net Carbs1.05g Protein1.08g.

LUNCH

221.   SALAD OF SESAME SALMON

Prep. Time: 5 min.   **Cooking time**: 20 min.   **Servings**: 2

Ingredient:
Salad
- One medium yellow pepper, chopped
- ¼ cup green onions, chopped
- One medium red pepper, chopped.
- One medium head lettuce, chopped
- Four tbsp. olive oil
- Two large (12-ounce each) salmon filets
- Two tbsp. coconut aminos
- One tsp. sesame oil

Dressing
- Five tbsp. coconut aminos
- One tsp. sesame oil
- Four tsp. olive oil

Directions:

1. Heat 3⁄4 of the olive oil in a medium heat pot for the salad. Add sesame oil, cocoon oil and amino liquids.
2. Cut your salmon into smaller pieces if necessary. (I halved the two filets to make four parts)
3. Put your salmon in the pan and give 5-7 min. of cooking time.
4. Flip over them and cook for another 5 min. When done, they should be light rose to white on the inside. Place your salmon in a salad bowl, while your salmon is cooking.
5. Mix the dressing ingredients together in a smaller bowl.
6. After the salmon are finished, put it on top of the salad, dress up and enjoy!

Nutrition: Calories 383 Fats 27.14g Net Carbs 7.33g Protein 24.3g

DINNER

222.   NACHO CHICKEN CASSEROLE

Prep. Time: 5 min.   **Cooking time:** 25 min.   **Servings:** 4

Ingredient:

- Salt and Pepper to Taste
- 1 1/2 tsp. Chili seasoning
- 1.75 lbs. Chicken Thighs, boneless skinless
- 4 oz. Cream Cheese
- 2 tbsp. Olive Oil
- 1 cup Green Chilies and Tomatoes
- 4 oz. Cheddar Cheese
- 1/4 cup Sour Cream
- 3 tbsp. Parmesan Cheese (~45g)
- One medium Jalapeño Pepper
- 16 oz. Frozen cauliflower, package

Directions:

1. Pre-heat 375F oven. Chop the chicken and season it, then cook in olive oil over medium to high until browned.
2. Add cream, sour cream and cheddar 3/4. Remove until melted and mixed together. Add tomatoes and chili green and mix together well. Add it all to a saucepan.
3. Frozen cauliflower microwave until cooked through. Using an immersion mixer to mix the rest of the cheese into a smooth potato. Saison to taste. Season to taste.
4. Cut jalapeño in pieces. Disseminate the cauliflower mixture over the top of the pot, then sprinkle the jalapeño pepper. Bake for fifteen-two min.

Nutrition: Calories 426 Fats 32.2g Net Carbs 4.3g Protein 30.8g.

DAY 2

BREAKFAST

223.   SAUSAGE GRAVY AND BISCUIT BAKE

Prep. Time: 10 min.   **Cooking time:** 30 min   **Servings:** 4

Ingredient:

- Two large egg whites
- One tsp. baking powder

Sausage Gravy:

- One tsp. xanthan gum
- 12 ounces ground pork breakfast sausage
- 1 cup almond flour
- Two tbsp. frozen butter

- ½ tsp. onion powder
- ½ cup half and half
- One tsp. black pepper
- ½ tsp. xanthan gum

- 1 ½ cups chicken broth
- ¼ tsp. salt, to taste

Directions:

1. Whisk the almond flour, baking powder and half a tsp. of xanthan gum together in a large cup.
2. Grate the frozen butter (or very cold). Mix with a

fork in the flour mix until it appears like coarse crumbs. Set aside. Set aside.

3. The egg whites beat in a separate medium-sized bowl to steep peaks. Fold the egg whites into the flour mix until they are only mixed with a rubber spatula.

4. Chill the biscuit mixture when making the gravy in the refrigerator.

5. Brown the sausage over medium heat in a large skillet. Remove the sausage from the paper towel plate to drain the excess grate and keep in the saucepan about a tbsp. of fat.

6. Switch the heat to medium-low and sprinkle one tsp. of xanthan gum into the grease.

7. Cook the xanthan gum about a min. until it is browned lightly. Chicken, onion powder and black pepper whisk in the stock. Bring to a frying pan and let it thicken about 5 min. Sample and add salt when necessary at this time.

8. Stir in half and half and boil until thick and fluffy, about 3 min more.

9. Remove the cooked sausage and remove from the sun. Preheat the oven to a temperature of 375 ° F.

10. Pour the sausage in an 8x8 saucepan.

11. Drop the biscuit mixture in tiny spoonful's over the gravy and spread as fairly as possible. The blend is going to be dense.

12. Bake until sweet, bubbled for 18-20 min., and the biscuits are baked and browned.

Nutrition Calories374.67 Fats33.21g Net Carbs4.75g Protein14.48g.

LUNCH

224. OVEN ROASTED CAPRESE SALAD

Prep. Time: 10 min. **Cooking time**: 30 min. **Servings**: 6

Ingredient:
- 3 cups grape tomatoes
- 4 cloves garlic, peeled
- 4 cups baby spinach
- 1 tbsp. avocado oil
- 1 tbsp. pesto
- 10 pieces' pearl size mozzarella balls
- ¼ cup basil, fresh
- 1 tbsp. brine, reserved from cheese

Directions:
1. Heat the oven to 400 ° F and prepare a foil bakery. Spread the skinned cloves of garlic and tomatoes uniformly.
2. Drizzle the tomatoes with avocado oil and mix them to coat. Bake for about 20-30 min or until the juices are loosened, and the tops are slightly brown.
3. Drain the mozzarella sauce, set aside 1 tbsp. and mix with pesto tbsp. of salt.
4. Take the tomatoes out of the oven and place the spinach in a vast portion dish.
5. Add the spinach and roast garlic to warm tomatoes and drizzle the pesto sauce.
6. Add mozzarella balls and new ripped basil leaves.

Nutrition: Calories190.75, Fats63.49g, Net Carbs4.58g, Protein7.79g.

DINNER

225. BUFFALO CHICKEN JALAPEÑO CASSEROLE

Prep. Time: 20 min. **Cooking time**: 55 min. **Servings**: 6

Ingredient:
- Six slices bacon
- boneless of 2-pound chicken thighs, (6-small)
- 12 ounces' cream cheese
- Three medium jalapeños
- 4 ounces shredded cheddar cheese
- ¼ cup mayonnaise
- ¼ cup Frank's Red Hot
- 2 ounces shredded mozzarella Cheese
- Salt and pepper to taste
- De-seed if you're not a spicy fan.

Directions:
1. De-bone the chicken thighs and pre-heat oven to 400F. Season with salt and pepper, then put on a cooling rack over a cookie sheet covered in foil. Bake thighs of chicken at 400F for 40 min.

2. After 20 min of your timer, start filling. Chop 6 bacon pieces and place them in a pot over medium heat. Upon most of the bacon is crisped, add jalapeños to the pot.

3. When they are soft and fried, add cream cheese, mayo and the red-hot franks to the pot. Mix together and taste the season.

4. Remove from the oven the chicken and let it cool slightly. Remove the skins from the chicken until they are cool enough.

5. Put the chicken into a dish of casserole and spread the cream cheese mixture over it and add the cheddar and mozzarella.

6. Bake at 400F for 10-15 min. Cook for 3-5 min. to complete. Optional: Top with additional jalapeños before broiling.

Nutrition: Calories 782 Fats 66.97g Net Carbs 4.59g Protein 38.61g.

DAY 3

BREAKFAST

226.   KETO COCONUT CREAM PIES

Prep. Time: 60 seconds   **Cooking time**: 5 min.   **Servings**: 2

Ingredient:

The Crust
- 4 tbsp. butter
- ¼ cup sugar substitute
- ½ cup almond flour
- ¼ cup unsweetened coconut flakes

The Custard
- 2 large egg yolks
- ¼ cup coconut flour
- 1 cup heavy whipping cream
- 1 tsp. vanilla extract
- ½ cup water
- ¼ cup sugar substitute

The Top
- 2 tbsp. sugar substitute
- 2-3 tbsp. unsweetened coconut flakes, toasted
- 1 cup heavy whipping cream
- 1 tsp. vanilla extract

Directions:

1. In a kettle, melt medium-low butter.
2. Stir in your sugar replacement until it dissolves in butter. Stir regularly. Mix your amber meal and coconut flakes until the mixture clumps easily together. Spoon the crust into a ramekin and flatten with a spoon.
3. Enable it to cool while making your custard
4. Heat your cream in a pot (I used the same pot as the crust). Separate the eggs and put them in a dish. It's time for the slurry!
5. Whisk your cocoa flour and the water. You should have a thick mixture of cocoa and egg.
6. Remove the vanilla from the stove to the milk.
7. Pour the slurry into the cream or spoon it.
8. Stir regularly with a whisk until the mixture thickens.
9. Let cool for about 5 min before spooning the custard on top of the crust into the ramekins.
10. Let the refrigerator set for at least one hour.
11. Heat your coconut flakes on a small pot to low. Stirring constantly. They are ready to toast when they are a perfect golden brown.
12. Remove the milk, vanilla and sugar in a big tub.
13. Beat the cream using a hand or stand mixer until it forms steep peaks.
14. Sprinkle the cream over the custard when ready to serve the custard and sprinkle the toasted coconut over it.

Nutrition: Calories 584 Net Carbs 7.25g Fats 57.33g Protein9.22g.

LUNCH

227.   KETO LEMON POPPY SEED SCONES

Prep. Time: 5 seconds   **Cooking time**: 30 min.   **Servings**: 2

Ingredient:
- 1 ½ cups almond flour
- 2 tbsp. coconut flour
- 1 tbsp. psyllium husk fiber
- 1/2 tsp. baking powder
- ¼ tsp. baking soda
- 1 tbsp. poppy seeds
- 4 tbsp. butter
- ¼ cup erythritol
- 2 large eggs

- ½ lemon, juice and zest
- 2 tbsp. erythritol, for sprinkling

Directions:

1. Then heat a 350F oven to a parchment paper baker. Combine almond flour, cocoa flour, psyllium husk fiber, baking powder and baking soda in a large mixing bowl. In cotton seeds, whisk until well mixed.
2. Break butter with a bell, pastry cutter or your hands into the dry ingredients to shape the dough.
3. In a separate cup, whisk eggs and sweetener together until sweetened.
4. Apply the sprinkling erythritol to the lemon on a tray. Mash sugar and zest together with a fork and set aside for dryness.
5. Break the lemon in half and squeeze the juice into the egg mixture, be careful not to get any seeds in the mixture.
6. In the dough, place the egg mixture and mix well.
7. Put the wet dough in the dome type on the prepared parchment.
8. Rate the wet dough carefully with a knife in 8 triangles and bake for 20 min.
9. Remove from an oven and cut into eight triangles. Sprinkle with lemon sugar and simmer for another 10 min.

Nutrition: Calories 206.8, Fat 18.5g Net Carbs 3.53g Protein 6.6g.

DINNER

228. LOW CARB HAMBURGER BUN

Prep. Time: 30 seconds **Cooking time:** 2 min. **Servings:** 1

Ingredient:

- 1 large egg
- 1 tbsp. melted butter
- 1 tbsp. chicken broth
- 1 tbsp. almond flour
- ¼ tsp. baking powder
- 1 tbsp. psyllium husk powder
- ¼ tsp. cream of tartar

Directions:

1. Crack the egg into a mug and put the melted butter into it. Remove well together until the eggs are lighter in color.
2. Apply the remaining ingredients and blend together thoroughly. You should have a slightly doughy substance.
3. Microwave for the 60-75 seconds, depending on the microwave wattage (it will buff in the mug, and reduce it greatly).
4. Cut in half and sprinkle with sugar.

Nutrition: Calories 248, Fats 19.77g, Net Carbs 3.01g, Protein 7.99g.

DAY 4

BREAKFAST

229. KETO AMARETTI COOKIES

Prep. Time: 5 min **Cooking time:** 16 min **Servings:** 10

Ingredient:

- 1 cup. Almond Flour
- 1 tbsp. Shredded Coconut
- 2 tbsp. Coconut Flour
- 1/4 tsp. Cinnamon
- 1/2 tsp. Baking Powder
- 1/2 cup Erythritol
- 1/2 tsp. Salt
- 2 large Eggs
- 1/2 tsp. Almond Extract
- 4 tbsp. Coconut Oil
- 1/2 tsp. Vanilla Extract
- 2 tbsp. Sugar-Free Jam

Directions:

1. Preheat your 350F oven. Combine all your dry ingredients and add the wet ingredients.
2. Shape your cookies on a bakery sheet lined with parchment paper. Use your finger to add an indent in the centre of each cookie.
3. Bake for about 16 min or until the cookies turn slightly golden. Let that cookie cool on a wire rack and make each indent with some sugar-free jam.
4. Sprinkle on top of each one some shredded coconut and enjoy!

Nutrition: Calories 89.38 Fats 8.11g Net Carbs 1.17g Protein 2.43g.

LUNCH

230. GRILLED SIRLOIN STEAK WITH CHIMICHURRI

Prep. Time: 10 Min   **Cooking Time**: 10 Min   **Servings**: 4

Ingredients

- 1.33 lbs. lean sirloin steak, trimmed (I recommend top sirloin)
- 1/2 tsp. black pepper
- 1 tsp. kosher salt
- 1/2 tsp. garlic powder
- 1/2 tsp. cumin
- 1 tbsp red wine vinegar
- 2 tbsp extra virgin olive oil
- 1 clove garlic, minced
- 2 tbsp parsley
- 2 tbsp cilantro
- 1 tbsp water
- 2 tbsp basil
- Salt and pepper

Directions:

1. Over medium heat preheat the grill or a grill pan.
2. In a blender or food processor, add red wine vinegar, olive oil, cilantro, basil, water, parsley, garlic, salt, and pepper. Mix until it forms a sauce, adding water if necessary. You can add red pepper flakes if you like spicy chimichurri.
3. Rub the salt, pepper, cumin, and garlic powder with the steak. Grill the steak to your desired doneness. Five min on each side for medium-rare, Get the steak removed and let it rest.
4. Thinly slice it on top of the grain and serve with chimichurri.

Nutrition Calories 280, Saturated Fat 6g, Polyunsaturated Fat 1g, Sodium 538mg, Total Carbohydrate 1g, Monounsaturated Fat 6g, Total Fat 19g, Sugars 0g, Cholesterol 87mg, Dietary Fiber 0g, Protein 25g.

DINNER

231.   SOY CHICKEN AND VEGETABLES

Prep. Time: 10 Min   **Cooking Time**: 25 Min   **Servings**: 4

Ingredients

- 1/4 cup low sodium soy sauce
- 1 tbsp rice wine vinegar
- 2 tbsp oyster sauce
- 1 tbsp sesame oil
- 1.33 lbs boneless skinless chicken thighs
- 2 cloves garlic, minced
- 1 cup mushrooms, halved
- 2 cups broccoli florets
- 1 cup sugar snap peas

Salt and pepper

- 1 tbsp freshly grated ginger
- 1 cup carrots, sliced
- 1 tsp. corn-starch
- 1 cup shelled edamame
- 2 green onions, sliced

Directions:

1. To 425 degrees, heat the oven. Sprinkle with cooking spray on a large baking sheet. First, cover the baking sheet in foil for easier clean-up and then spray. In a small cup, add the soya sauce, rice vinegar, oyster sauce, corn-starch, sesame oil, garlic, and ginger and stir together.
2. On both sides, season the chicken with pepper. Place and drizzle with around half the soy mixture on the baking sheet so that both sides are coated. Put the mixture in the oven and cook for ten min.
3. Remove it from the oven and spread the vegetables around the chicken on the baking sheet. Drizzle the remaining soy mixture with it. Return to the oven and cook for 10-15 min until the chicken is cooked and the vegetables are crisp and tender.

Nutrition: Calories 320, Sugars 4g, Monounsaturated Fat 3g, Saturated Fat 2g, Dietary Fiber 6g, Polyunsaturated Fat 3g, Total Fat 11g, Total Carbohydrate 17g, Cholesterol 131mg, Sodium 1048mg, Protein 39g.

DAY 5

BREAKFAST

232.   KETO WHIPPED CREAM

Prep. Time: 60 seconds   **Cooking time**: 5 min   **Servings**: 2

Ingredient:

- 1 cup heavy cream, chilled well
- 1 tsp. vanilla extract
- 1 tbsp. erythritol, powdered

Directions:

1. Using a spice grinder or small blender to powder erythritol. Set aside the remaining ingredients.
2. Pour in a large, dry blender bowl with cold heavy cream. When washed beforehand, make sure all water is wiped from the blending bowl as only a small quantity of water can ruin whipped cream.
3. Start mixing the cream slowly with a hand mixer.

Step up as the cream thickens so as not to sprinkle the cream.

4. Add powdered erythritol and vanilla extract after approximately 60 seconds of whipping.

5. Continue to whip to form medium peaks. The peaks on your beaters should be notified when they are taken out of the cream.

6. Move the cream to a bowl to serve your favourite dish. You can save 2-3 days in the fridge in an airtight jar.

Nutrition: 103 Calories, 0.9g Net Carbs, 10.8g Fats, 0.9g Protein.

LUNCH

233. KALE SOUP AND SAUSAGE

Prep. Time: 10 min   **Cooking time**: 25 min   **Servings**: 2

Ingredient:

- 1 Tbsp. butter
- 1 lb. sweet Italian sausage, ground
- One medium carrot, peeled and diced
- One medium yellow onion, chopped
- 2 tbsp. red wine vinegar
- Two cloves garlic, crushed
- 1 tsp. dried basil
- 1 tsp. dried oregano
- ¼ – ½ tsp. crushed red pepper flakes
- 1 tsp. dried rubbed sage
- 1 cup heavy whipping cream
- 4 cups low-sodium chicken broth
- 3 cups kale, chopped
- ½ medium head cauliflower, cut into small florets
- ½ tsp. freshly ground black pepper
- ½ – 1 tsp. sea salt, or to taste

Directions:

1. Heat a large casserole or Netherlands oven over medium heat. Attach ground sausage and split the beef. Cook and stir it occasionally, for 5 min, until browned and cooked.

2. Remove cooked sausage using a slotted spoon and make the drainage on a sheet covered with paper towels. Drippings discard but do not wash the pan.

3. Melt medium heat butter. Attach onion and carrot when bubbling subsides. Cook until the onion becomes brown and translucent on the outside.

4. Mix garlic into the mixture of onion and carrot. Cook one min. Cook one min. Add vinegar of red wine and cook until sip, scrap browned bits for approximately 1 min.

5. Remove the flakes of oregano, basil, wise and red pepper. Pour in heavy cream and stock. Increase medium-high sun. When the soup cooks, add colic and turn heat to medium-low. Simmer uncovered for about ten min, until cauliflower is fork-tender. Stir in the cooked sausage and kale. Cook for like 2 min, and/or till the sausage and kale wilts are restored.

6. Season with salt and pepper to taste. The amount of salt required can vary because of variations in broth marks.

Nutrition: Calories 298 Fats 24g Net Carbs 6g Protein 16g

DINNER

234. LOW CARB CORNED BEEF CABBAGE ROLLS

Prep. Time: 30 min   **Cooking time**: 6 hours 5min   **Servings**: 4

Ingredient:

- pounds corned beef
- 1 medium onion
- 15 large savoy cabbage leaves
- 1 large lemon
- ¼ cup white wine
- 1 large bay leaf
- ¼ cup coffee
- 1 tbsp. rendered bacon fat
- 1 tbsp. NOW Erythritol
- 1 tbsp. brown mustard
- 2 tsp. kosher salt
- 1 tsp. whole peppercorns
- 2 tsp. Worcestershire
- 1 tsp. mustard seeds
- ¼ tsp. cloves
- ½ tsp. red pepper flakes
- ¼ tsp. allspice

Directions:

1. Connect to the slow cooker the corned beef, liquids and spices. Let this cook on low for 6 hours.

2. Put a pot of water to a boil when it is about to be taken.

3. Add the 15 cod leaves plus 1 sliced onion for 2-3 min to the boiling water.

4. Remove the cod from the water and blanch for 3-4 min in ice water. Continue to boil in the water the onion.

5. Dry chops, cut meat, apply ointments and roll fillings into the chops.

6. Optional: Serve with a new lemon squeeze!

Nutrition: Calories481.4 Fats25.38g Net Carbs4.2g Protein34.87g

DAY 6

BREAKFAST

235.   GRILLED BUFFALO CHICKEN SANDWICHES

Prep. Time: 5 Min   **Cooking Time**: 15 Min   **Servings**: 4

Ingredients

- 1 lb. boneless skinless chicken breasts
- Cooking spray
- 1 tsp. paprika
- 1/4 cup blue cheese
- 1 tsp. chili powder
- 1/4 cup buffalo sauce
- Salt and pepper
- 1/4 cup nonfat plain Greek yogurt
- 4 tsp. butter
- 4 reduced calorie hamburger buns

Directions:

1. Cut the chicken into thinner cutlets or pound it. Season with paprika, chili powder, salt, and pepper and sprinkle with cooking spray.
2. Over medium-high heat, heat a grill, grill pan, or skillet. If required, sprinkle with cooking spray. Cook the chicken on each side for 3-4 min or until it has cooked through.
3. Meanwhile, yogurt and blue cheese are mixed together to produce a burger sauce. With salt and pepper, season. The butter is melted and stirred into the buffalo sauce. Toss this mixture with the cooked chicken breasts.
4. Put the sandwiches together and add lettuce, tomatoes, onions, and any other toppings that you want.

Nutrition: Calories 285, Saturated Fat 4g, Cholesterol 72mg, Monounsaturated Fat 0g, Total Fat 8g, Total Carbohydrate 19g, Sugars 3g, Sodium 403mg, Polyunsaturated Fat 0g, Dietary Fiber 3g, Protein 31g.

LUNCH

236.   GRILLED PORK CHOPS WITH PEACH SALSA

Prep. Time: 10 Min   **Cooking Time**: 15 Min   **Servings**: 4

Ingredients

- 1.33 lbs. boneless lean center cut pork chops
- 1 tsp. chili powder (or more)
- 2 tbsp. olive oil, divided
- Salt and pepper
- 1/2 tsp. salt
- 2 peaches, chopped
- 1/2 tsp. pepper
- 2 tbsp. cilantro
- 1/4 red onion, chopped
- 1 tbsp. lime juice

Directions:

1. Preheat to medium-high heat on the grill or a grill pan. You may use the broiler as well.
2. Brush the olive oil with the pork chops and sprinkle on both sides with chili powder, salt, and pepper.
3. Grill on each side for 4-5 min (or to the desired level). Let yourself rest for 5 min. Place on a baking sheet on a wire rack to broil and broil for 4-5 min per side.
4. Toss the lime juice, peaches, cilantro, onion, and olive oil together to make the salsa: season with salt and pepper season. Over pork, serve. Grill the peaches before making the salsa for a fun twist.

Nutrition: Calories 287, Monounsaturated Fat 2g, Saturated Fat 3g, Total Carbohydrate 9g, Polyunsaturated Fat 1g, Total Fat 12g, Sodium 381mg, Cholesterol 100mg, Sugars 7g, Dietary Fiber 1g, Protein 35g.

DINNER

237.   PASTA WITH FRESH TOMATO SAUCE

Prep. Time: 40 Min   **Cooking Time**: 10 Min   **Servings**: 4

Ingredients

- 1 tsp. thyme
- 2 lbs. tomatoes, diced (about ½ inch.)
- 1/2 cup fresh basil (or parsley)
- 2 tbsp. olive oil
- 8 oz. high fiber pasta
- 2 tbsp. balsamic vinegar
- Salt and pepper
- 2 garlic cloves, minced

Directions:

1. Toss together the tomatoes, olive oil, basil (or parsley), thyme, vinegar, garlic, salt, and pepper. Let it sit for 30 min at room temperature (up to 4 hours.)
2. Cook the pasta according to package instructions when ready to eat. Toss in the warm tomato pasta and eat.

Nutrition: Calories 281, Saturated Fat 1g, Polyunsaturated Fat 0g, Total Fat 13g, Cholesterol 0mg, Dietary Fiber 9g, Sodium 14mg, Total Carbohydrate 52g, Sugars 9g, Monounsaturated Fat 0g, Protein 8g.

DAY 7

BREAKFAST

238.   BACON CRUSTED FRITTATA MUFFINS

Prep. Time: 5 min   **Cooking time:** 30 min   **Servings:** 5

Ingredient:

- ½ tsp. onion powder
- 18 slices bacon
- ½ tsp. cayenne pepper
- 7 large eggs
- 1 cup cheddar cheese
- 4 tbsp. heavy whipping cream
- ½ tsp. ground black pepper
- ½ tsp. celery salt

Directions:

1. Preheat your 375F oven.
2. Break your bacon pieces in half and mold them in a cupcake bowl around the outsides and underneath of each well. You can use roughly 2 bacon slices per well, often more to fill in excess gaps.
3. Bake the bacon baskets 15 min in the oven before cooking. While the bacon is being fried, whisk some eggs, cream and spices together. Feel free to add some additional fresh herbs.
4. Put 1-2 dc. Cheddar cheese at the base of any frittata bacon. Put approximately 1/4 of an egg mixture in any bacon mold and do your best not to leave out any egg. Put them in the oven for a further 12-15 min or until they begin browning on top.
5. Take off the oven, let it cool. Serve or shop later!

Nutrition: Calories 467.57 Net Carbs 2.23g Fats 41.83g Protein 19.35g.

LUNCH

239.   GRILLED CHICKEN WITH PEACH CUCUMBER SALSA

Prep. Time: 10 Min   **Cooking Time:** 10 Min   **Servings:** 4

Ingredients

- 1.33 lbs. boneless skinless chicken breast
- 1 tbsp. honey (leave out for Low Carb, Paleo, Whole30)
- 1 tbsp. olive oil
- 1 tsp. cumin
- 1 tbsp. soy sauce
- 2 peaches, diced
- 1/2 tsp. pepper
- 1/4 cup red onion, diced
- 2 Persian cucumbers, diced
- 1 tbsp. lime juice
- 1/4 cup cilantro, minced
- 1 tbsp. rice wine vinegar

Directions:

1. Put the olive oil, the honey, the soy sauce, the cumin and the pepper together. With this mixture, clean the chicken.
2. Mix the peaches, the cucumber, the red onion, the lime juice, the olive oil, and the rice vinegar. With salt and pepper, season.
3. On a medium hot grill, grill the chicken for 3-5 min on each side, depending on the thickness of your chicken. After grill marks emerge, flip it and the chicken is quickly removed from the grill.
4. With the cucumber salsa and peach on top, serve the chicken.

Nutrition: Calories 265, Saturated Fat 2g, Polyunsaturated Fat 0g, Cholesterol 243mg, Total Fat 10g, Total Carbohydrate 11g, Sodium 556mg, Dietary Fiber 2g, Sugars 8g, Monounsaturated Fat 0g, Protein 34g.

DINNER

240.   BAKED SCAMPI

Prep time: 30 min   **Cook time:** 15 min   **Servings** 4

Ingredients

- 1 tbsp. fresh lemon juice
- 1 tbsp. garlic, chopped
- 1 tbsp. fresh parsley, chopped
- 2 tbsp. prepared Dijon mustard
- 2 pounds (907 g) raw shrimp,
- medium, shelled, deveined, with tails attached
- 1 cup butter

Directions:

1. Start by preheating the oven to 450°F (235°C).
2. Mix the lemon juice, butter, garlic, parsley and mustard in a small saucepan over moderate heat until the butter melts.
3. In a baking dish, place the shrimp, then pour over the butter mixture.
4. Arrange the dish in the preheated oven and bake for 13 min or until the shrimp are easily flaked with a fork. Remove the baking pan from the oven and serve warm.

Nutrition: Calories: 420 Total Fat: 32.9g Carbs: 1.7g Protein: 29.7g Cholesterol: 320mg Sodium: 681mg

WEEK 2

DAY 1

BREAKFAST

241.   CHORIZO BREAKFAST

Prep Time: 10 min   **Cooking Time**: 12 min   **Servings**: 2

Ingredients

- 1 tbsp. olive oil
- ½ cup diced red pepper
- ½ cup diced yellow onion
- 4 ounces chorizo sausage
- 2 large eggs
- Salt and pepper
- 2 slices thick-cut bacon, cooked

Directions:

1. Preheat the oven to 350°F and lightly grease two ramekins.
2. Heat the oil in a skillet over medium-high heat.
3. Add the peppers and onions and cook for 4 to 5 min until browned.
4. Divide the vegetable mixture between the two ramekins.
5. Chop the chorizo and divide between the ramekins.
6. Crack an egg into each ramekin and season with salt and pepper, to taste.
7. Bake for 10 to 12 min until the egg is set to the desired level.
8. Crumble the bacon over top and serve hot.

Nutrition: Calories 450 Fat 36 g Net Carb 4.5 g Total Carbs: 5.5 g Fiber: 1 g Protein 25 g

LUNCH

242.   PORK LETTUCE WRAPS

Prep Time: 10 min   **Cooking Time**: 15 min   **Servings**: 2

Ingredients

- 1 tbsp. olive oil
- ¼ cup diced yellow onion
- ¼ cup diced green pepper
- 2 tbsp. diced celery
- 6 ounces ground pork
- ¼ teaspoon onion powder
- ¼ tsp. garlic powder
- 2 tbsp. soy sauce
- 1 tsp. sesame oil
- 4 leaves butter lettuce, separated
- 1 tbsp. toasted sesame seeds

Directions:

1. Heat the oil in a skillet over medium heat.
2. Add the onions, peppers, and celery and sauté for 5 min until tender.
3. Stir in the pork and cook until just browned.
4. Add the onion powder and garlic powder, then stir in the soy sauce and sesame oil.
5. Season with salt and pepper to taste, then remove from heat.
6. Place the lettuce leaves on a plate and spoon the pork mixture evenly into them.
7. Sprinkle with sesame seeds to serve.

Nutrition: Calories 500 Fat 29 g Net Carb 7.5 g Total Carbs: 10.5 g Fiber: 3 g Protein 49 g

DINNER

243.   AVOCADO LIME SALMON

Prep Time: 15 min   **Cooking Time**: 15 min   **Servings**: 2

Ingredients

- 100 grams chopped cauliflower
- 1 large avocado
- 1 tbsp. fresh lime juice
- 2 tbsp. diced red onion
- 2 tbsp. olive oil
- 2 (6-ounce) boneless salmon fillets
- Salt and pepper

Directions:

1. Place the cauliflower in a food processor and pulse into rice-like grains.
2. Grease a skillet with cooking spray and heat over medium heat.
3. Add the cauliflower rice and cook, covered, for 8 min until tender. Set aside.
4. Combine the avocado, lime juice, and red onion in a food processor and blend smooth.
5. Heat the oil in a large skillet over medium-high heat.
6. Season the salmon with salt and pepper, then add to the skillet skin-side down.
7. Cook for 4 to 5 min until seared, then flip and cook for another 4 to 5 min.
8. Serve the salmon over a bed of cauliflower rice topped with the avocado cream.

Nutrition: Calories 570 Fat 44 g Net Carb 4 g Total Carbs: 12 g Fiber: 8 g Protein 36 g

DAY 2

BREAKFAST

244.   LOW-CARB BREAKFAST EGG MUFFINS WITH SAUSAGE GRAVY

Prep Time: 15 min   **Cooking Time**: 35 min   **Servings**: 6

Ingredients

For the muffins:

- 12 large eggs
- Sea salt
- Black pepper
- 1 pound thin shaved deli ham
- 4 ounces shredded mozzarella cheese
- 4 ounces grated parmesan cheese
- Low-carb sausage gravy

For the gravy:

- 1/2 ground pork sausage
- 8 ounces softened cream cheese
- 3/4 cups beef broth
- Sea salt
- Black pepper

Directions:

1. Prepare the eggs and gravy.
2. Whisk eggs together with salt and pepper to taste.
3. Cook the sausage over medium heat until thoroughly cooked through. Add in the cream cheese and the broth and stirring constantly, cook until the mixture comes to a soft simmer and thickens.
4. Then reduce the heat to medium-low, still stirring constantly and simmer for 2 more min.
5. Season to taste with salt and pepper.
6. Set mixture aside.
7. Preheat oven to 325°F.

Assemble the muffins:

1. Place two pieces of ham in the bottom of each muffin cup, careful to overlap and try and cover the whole surface. Evenly divide sausage gravy between each muffin.
2. Pour eggs into each muffin, dividing the mixture evenly.
3. Top each muffin with equal parts of the two types of cheeses.
4. Bake for approximately 30-40 min or until muffin is firm and cheese is melted.

Nutrition: Calories 607 Fat 46 g Net Carb 3 g Total Carbs: 6 g Fiber: 3 g Protein 42 g

LUNCH

245.   SPICED PUMPKIN SOUP

Prep Time: 15 min   **Cooking Time**: 40 min   **Servings**: 3

Ingredients

- 2 tbsp. unsalted butter
- 1 small yellow onion, chopped
- 2 cloves minced garlic
- 1 teaspoon minced ginger
- ½ teaspoon ground cinnamon
- ¼ teaspoon ground nutmeg
- Salt and pepper, to taste
- ½ cup pumpkin puree
- 1 cup chicken broth
- 3 slices thick-cut bacon
- ¼ cup heavy cream

Directions:

1. Melt the butter in a large saucepan over medium heat.
2. Add the onions, garlic, and ginger and cook for 3 to 4 min until the onions are translucent.
3. Stir in the spices and cook for 1 min until fragrant. Season with salt and pepper.
4. Add the pumpkin puree and chicken broth, then bring to a boil.
5. Reduce heat and simmer for 20 min, then remove from heat.
6. Puree the soup using an immersion blender, then return to heat and simmer for 20 min.
7. Cook the bacon in a skillet until crisp, then remove to paper towels to drain.
8. Add the bacon fat to the soup along with the heavy cream. Crumble the bacon over top to serve.

Nutrition: Calories 250 Fat 20 g Net Carb 6 g Total Carbs: 8 g Fiber: 2 g Protein 0 g

DINNER

246. EASY CHICKEN WITH SPINACH AND BACON

Prep Time: 10 min   **Cooking Time:** 20 min   **Servings:** 2

Ingredients

- 1 chicken breast, boiled
- 1 slice bacon, chopped
- 2 tbsp butter
- 1/2 cup spinach, chopped
- 1 tbsp onion in slices
- 2 tbsp cream cheese
- 1 tsp Italian seasoning
- 1 tsp salt
- 1/2 tsp black pepper

Directions:

1. First, let the chicken boil in hot water. Afterwards, shred it with a fork or with your hands. Set aside.
2. Pan fry the chopped bacon in melted butter. When the bacon starts producing fats, gently drop the shredded chicken in and cook for 2-3 min.
3. Toss in the spinach and onion into the pan. Leave to soften the vegetables.
4. Mix in the cream cheese and stir continuously to blend the ingredients. Add more flavor with the Italian seasoning, pepper, and salt.
5. Transfer to a serving plate and enjoy your meal.

Nutrition: Calories 383 Fat 3.2 g Net Carb 0.9 g Total Carbs: 1.2 g Fiber: 0.3 g Protein 40.3 g

DAY 3

BREAKFAST

247. BAKED EGGS IN AVOCADO

Prep Time: 5 min   **Cooking Time:** 15 min   **Servings:** 3

Ingredients

- 1 medium avocado
- 2 tbsp. lime juice
- 2 large eggs
- Salt and pepper
- 2 tbsp. shredded cheddar cheese

Directions:

1. Preheat the oven to 450°F and cut the avocado in half. Scoop out some of the flesh from the middle of each avocado half.
2. Place the avocado halves upright in a baking dish and brush with lime juice.
3. Crack an egg into each and season with salt and pepper.
4. Bake for 10 min, then sprinkle with cheese.
5. Let the eggs bake for another 2 to 3 min until the cheese is melted. Serve hot.

Nutrition: Calories 610 Fat 54 g Net Carb 4.5 g Total Carbs: 18 g Fiber: 13.5 g Protein 20 g

LUNCH

248.   EASY BEEF CURRY

Prep Time: 20 min   **Cooking Time**: 40 min   **Servings**: 3

Ingredients

- 1 medium yellow onion, chopped
- 1 tbsp. minced garlic
- 1 tbsp. grated ginger
- 1 ¼ cups canned coconut milk
- 1 pound beef chuck, chopped
- 2 tbsp. curry powder
- 1 tsp. salt
- ½ cup fresh chopped cilantro

Directions:

1. Combine the onion, garlic, and ginger in a food processor and blend into a paste.
2. Transfer the paste to a saucepan and cook for 3 min on medium heat.
3. Stir in the coconut milk, then simmer gently for 10 min.
4. Add the chopped beef along with the curry powder and salt. Stir well then simmer, covered, for 20 min. Remove the lid and simmer for another 20 min until the beef is cooked through.
5. Adjust seasoning to taste and garnish with fresh chopped cilantro.

Nutrition: Calories 550 Fat 34 g Net Carb 9 g Total Carbs: 14 g Fiber: 5 g Protein 50 g

DINNER

249.   ROSEMARY ROASTED CHICKEN AND VEGGIES

Prep Time: 15 min   **Cooking Time**: 35 min   **Servings**: 2

Ingredients

- 4 deboned chicken thighs
- Salt and pepper
- 1 small zucchini, sliced
- 2 small carrots, peeled and sliced
- 1 small parsnip, peeled and sliced
- 2 cloves garlic, sliced
- 3 tbsp. olive oil
- 1 tbsp. balsamic vinegar
- 2 tsp. fresh chopped rosemary

Directions:

1. Preheat the oven to 350°F and lightly grease a small rimmed baking sheet with cooking spray.
2. Place the chicken thighs on the baking sheet and season with salt and pepper.
3. Arrange the veggies around the chicken then sprinkle with sliced garlic.
4. Whisk together the remaining ingredients then drizzle over the chicken and veggies.
5. Bake for 30 min then broil for 3 to 5 min until the skins are crisp.

Nutrition Calories 540 Fat 40.5 g Net Carb 8.5 g Total Carbs: 12 g Fiber: 3.5 g Protein 33 g

DAY 4

BREAKFAST

250.   LEMON POPPY RICOTTA PANCAKES

Prep Time: 10 min   **Cooking Time**: 20 min   **Servings**: 2

Ingredients

- 1 large lemon, juiced and zested
- 6 ounces whole milk ricotta
- 3 large eggs
- 10 to 12 drops liquid stevia
- ¼ cup almond flour
- 1 scoop egg white protein powder
- 1 tbsp. poppy seeds
- ¾ teaspoons baking powder
- ¼ cup powdered erythritol
- 1 tbsp. heavy cream

Directions:

1. Combine the ricotta, eggs, and liquid stevia in a food processor with half the lemon juice and the lemon zest—blend well, then pour into a bowl.
2. Whisk in the almond flour, protein powder, poppy seeds, baking powder, and a pinch of salt.
3. Heat a large nonstick pan over medium heat.

4. Spoon the batter into the pan, using about ¼ cup per pancake.

5. Cook the pancakes until bubbles form on the surface of the batter, then flip them. Let the pancakes cook until the bottom is browned, then remove to a plate. Repeat with the remaining batter.

6. Whisk together the heavy cream, powdered erythritol, and reserved lemon juice and zest.

7. Serve the pancakes hot, drizzled with the lemon glaze.

Nutrition: Calories 370 Fat 26 g Net Carb 5.5 g Total Carbs: 6.5 g Fiber: 1 g Protein 29.5g

LUNCH

251. KETO BACON CHEESEBURGER WITH MUSHROOMS

Prep Time: 5 min   **Cooking Time**: 15 min   **Servings**: 4

Ingredients

- 1 lb ground beef
- 4 slices bacon
- 1 small egg
- 1 tbsp almond flour
- 1 tsp cumin
- 1/2 cup sliced mushrooms
- 1 tsp garlic powder
- 1 tsp onion powder
- 8 cheddar cheese thin slices
- Salt
- 1 tsp black pepper

Directions:

1. Season the ground beef with all of the condiments. Crack the egg into the beef and throw in the almond flour as well. Knead until well combined. Mold into 4 meatballs. Create the hollow shape of the meatballs with a soda can. Using your hands, shape the beef to form a cup before removing the can.

2. Fill the molded beef with mushroom. Wrap a slice of bacon around the sides of the cup.

3. Lay a slice of cheese on the surface of the hamburger to cover the mushroom. Leave in the 300°F oven for 10 min. Remove once the meat is cooked.

4. Lay another slice of cheese on top and rebake for an additional 5 min, enough to melt the cheese.

5. Serve and enjoy!

Nutrition: Calories 627 Fat 50.7 g Net Carb 2.2 g Total Carbs: 3 g Fiber: 0.8 g Protein 39.6g

DINNER

252. STUFFED CHICKEN BREASTS

Prep Time: 10 min   **Cooking Time**: 30 min   **Servings**: 3

Ingredients

- 1.5 lb chicken breast, approx. 3 pcs
- 1 cup chopped spinach fresh
- 1/2 cup cherry tomatoes
- 1 garlic clove
- 6 tbsp shredded cheese
- 2 tbsp olive oil
- 1/2 cup Rao's homemade tomato basil sauce (optional)

Directions:

1. Prepare all ingredients.

2. Add one tbsp of olive oil in a skillet, add spinach, quartet cherry tomatoes, and chopped garlic. Cook it until spinach is soft.

3. Make pockets in chicken breasts. Salt, pepper, you can add Mediterranean dry herbs (basil, oregano). I had three chicken breasts so I first stuffed each with one tbsp of cheese and then cooked greens. Close cuts with wooden toothpicks.

4. Brown chicken in the skillet on both sides (don't cook it) then transfer into a deep tray with the remaining tbsp of olive oil.

5. Distribute sauce evenly on top of the chicken. Cover with foil. Preheat oven to 375°F. Cook till it's done. As a final step sprinkle remaining cheese on top of the chicken, send it back to oven for a few min for cheese to melt.

6. Enjoy.

Nutrition: Calories 417 Fat 17.9 g Net Carb 2.6 g Total Carbs: 3.6 g Fiber: 1 g Protein 58.7g

DAY 5

BREAKFAST

253.   EGG WITH BLUEBERRIES AND CINNAMON

Prep Time: 5 min   **Cooking Time**: 20 min   **Servings**: 4

Ingredients

- 6 large eggs
- 2 tbsp softened butter
- 1 tsp vanilla
- 1/2 cup blueberries (or 1/4 cup, depending upon taste)
- 1/2 tsp cinnamon (you could probably double this if you like cinnamon)
- 1 tbsp coconut oil

Directions:

1. Preheat oven to 375°F. In an 8" – 9" cast iron skillet (or any oven-proof skillet), heat coconut oil over medium heat.
2. In a medium bowl beat eggs, butter, cinnamon, and vanilla together with a hand mixer until combined and fluffy (about 1-2 min).
3. Pour egg mixture into heated pan and allow bottom to cook slightly (about 2 min). Gently drop blueberries into egg mixture and place pan in oven. Cook for 15-20 or until cooked through and browned on top (but not burned).
4. Remove from oven and allow to cool slightly.

Nutrition: Calories 188 Fat 15 g Net Carb 1 g Total Carbs: 4 g Fiber: 3 g Protein 8 g

LUNCH

254.   LETTUCE ROLLS WITH GROUND BEEF

Prep Time: 10 min   **Cooking Time**: 15 min   **Servings**: 4

Ingredients

- 4 lettuce leaves
- ½ lb ground beef
- 1 tbsp olive oil
- 2 tbsp chopped onion
- 1 small tomato, chopped
- ½ tsp paprika
- 1 small avocado, chopped
- 2 tbsp sour cream
- ½ tsp salt
- ½ tsp black pepper

Directions:

1. In a hot frying pan with a tbsp of olive oil, sauté the onion and tomato. Gently plop the beef into the sautéed onion and tomato. Season with pepper, salt, paprika, and any other spice of your choice. Sear for 7-10 min over medium-high heat.
2. Lay the lettuce leaf on a flat board. Scoop out some of the cooked beef and place this on one side of the leaf. Top with avocado and sour cream. Roll the leaf firmly. Repeat until all of the ingredients are used up. Transfer to a plate and enjoy!

Nutrition: Calories 127 Fat 8.5 g Net Carb 1.4 g Total Carbs: 2.1 g Fiber: 0.7 g Protein 10.6 g

DINNER

255.   HOMEMADE SAGE SAUSAGE PATTIES

Prep. Time: 25 min.   **Cooking Time**: 15 min   **Servings**: 8

Ingredients

- 1 pound ground pork
- 3/4 cup shredded cheddar cheese
- 1/4 cup buttermilk
- 1 tbsp. finely chopped onion
- 2 teaspoons rubbed sage
- 3/4 teaspoon salt
- 3/4 teaspoon pepper
- 1/8 teaspoon garlic powder
- 1/8 teaspoon dried oregano

Directions:

1. In a bowl, combine all ingredients, mixing lightly but thoroughly. Shape into eight 1/2-inch-thick patties. Refrigerate 1 hour.
2. In a large cast-iron or other heavy skillet, cook patties over medium heat until a thermometer reads 160° 6-8 min on each side.

Nutrition: Calories 162 Fat 11 g Carbohydrates: 1 g Protein 13 g

DAY 6

BREAKFAST
256.   SWEET BLUEBERRY COCONUT PORRIDGE
Prep Time: 5 min   **Cooking Time**: 15 min   **Servings**: 2
Ingredients
- 1 cup unsweetened almond milk
- ¼ cup canned coconut milk
- ¼ cup coconut flour
- ¼ cup ground flaxseed
- 1 tsp. ground cinnamon
- ¼ teaspoon ground nutmeg
- Pinch salt
- 60 grams fresh blueberries
- ¼ cup shaved coconut

Directions:
1. Warm the almond milk and coconut milk in a saucepan over low heat. Whisk in the coconut flour, flaxseed, cinnamon, nutmeg, and salt. Turn up the heat and cook until the mixture bubbles.
2. Stir in the sweetener and vanilla extract, then cook until thickened to the desired level.
3. Spoon into two bowls and top with blueberries and shaved coconut.

Nutrition: Calories 390 Fat 22 g Net Carb 15 g Total Carbs: 37 g Fiber: 22 g Protein 10 g

LUNCH
257.   STUFFED JALAPENO PEPPERS WITH GROUND BEEF
Prep Time: 15 min   **Cooking Time**: 30 min   **Servings**: 6
Ingredients
- 6 large jalapeños
- 1 tbsp olive oil
- ½ lb ground beef
- 2 tbsp chopped onion
- 1 small tomato, chopped
- 2 oz grated mozzarella cheese
- ½ tsp salt
- ½ tsp black pepper

Directions:
1. While preparing the dish, let the oven preheat at 350°F. Heat the olive oil in a frying pan. Sauté the beef in the pan together with the onion and chopped tomato. Add salt and pepper to taste. Leave to cook for approximately 15 min.
2. Slice the jalapeños into two pieces. Empty the insides of the slices by discarding the seeds and the veins.
3. Stuff about a tbsp. ful of the cooked beef in the empty jalapeño halves. Sprinkle mozzarella cheese on the surface. Arrange the filled peppers on a baking sheet and cook in the oven for 15 min. Wait till the cheese browns.
4. Serve on a plate and enjoy!

Nutrition: Calories 127 Fat 8.5 g Net Carb 1.4 g Total Carbs: 2.1 g Fiber: 0.7 g Protein 10.6 g

DINNER
258.   SAUTEED SAUSAGE WITH GREEN BEANS
Prep Time: 15 min   **Cooking Time**: 15 min   **Servings**: 3
Ingredients
- 300 g pork sausage
- 1/2 cup green beans
- 1/2 onion, sliced
- 1/2 tbsp olive oil
- 2 tbsp sour cream
- Salt and pepper, to taste

Directions:
1. Chop off both tips of the green beans then slice into two. Put aside.
2. Chop the sausage links into bite-sized chunks as well. Reserve in a bowl. For easy chopping, refrigerate the sausage for around 15 min before cutting.
3. Preheat a skillet then pour the oil into heat. Sear the sausage chunks for 5 min.
4. Once brown, toss in the onion and chopped green beans. Sauté for 4-5 min more.
5. Gently pour in the cream. Season with pepper and salt. Fold the mix with a spatula to

incorporate all the ingredients together. Leave for an additional 3 min before turning off the heat.

6. Serve in a dish and enjoy warm.

Nutrition: Calories 369 Fat 32.6 g Net Carb 3.6 g Total Carbs: 4.5 g Fiber: 0.9 g Protein 15 g

DAY 7

BREAKFAST

259. LOW-CARB BREAKFAST QUICHE

Prep Time: 15 min   **Cooking Time**: 55 min   **Servings**: 4

Ingredients
- 1 lb ground Italian sausage
- 1.5 cups shredded cheddar cheese
- 8 large eggs
- 1 tbsp ranch seasoning
- 1 cup sour cream

Directions:
1. Preheat oven to 350°F.
2. In an oven-safe skillet, brown ground sausage and drain the grease.
3. In a large bowl, whisk together egg, sour cream, and ranch seasoning. You may want to use a hand mixer.
4. Mix in cheddar cheese.
5. Pour egg mixture into pan and stir until everything is fully blended.
6. Cover with foil and bake for 30 min.
7. Remove foil and bake for another 25 min or until golden brown.

Nutrition: Calories 551 Fat 46 g Net Carb 3 g Total Carbs: 6 g Fiber: 3 g Protein 26 g

LUNCH

260. BACON WRAPPED ASPARAGUS

Prep Time: 5 min   **Cooking Time**: 20 min   **Servings**: 2

Ingredients
- 12 spear fresh asparagus, medium-sized
- 2 tbsp olive oil
- 6 slices bacon
- Salt and black pepper, to taste

Directions:
1. Set the oven to 350°F to preheat. After rinsing the asparagus with water, chop off the tough parts of the stem.
2. Drizzle olive oil on the asparagus spears. Salt and pepper to enhance the flavor. Wrap half a strip of bacon around each asparagus. Repeat until all the ingredients are used up.
3. Arrange the wrapped asparagus on a baking sheet in a way that they don't overlap. Leave in the oven for 20 min. Wait till the vegetable is tender.
4. Transfer to a plate. Best served warm.

Nutrition: Calories 565 Fat 54.6 g Net Carb 2.8 g Total Carbs: 4.8 g Fiber: 2 g Protein 15 g

DINNER

261. LAMB CHOPS WITH ROSEMARY AND GARLIC

Prep Time: 35 min   **Cooking Time**: 15 min   **Servings**: 2

Ingredients
- 1 tbsp. coconut oil, melted
- 1 tsp. fresh chopped rosemary
- 1 clove garlic, minced
- 2 bone-in lamb chops (about 6 ounces meat)
- 1 tbsp. butter
- Salt and pepper
- ¼ pound fresh asparagus, trimmed
- 1 tbsp. olive oil

Directions:
1. Combine the coconut oil, rosemary, and garlic in a shallow dish. Add the lamb chops then turn to coat – let marinate in the fridge overnight. Let the lamb rest at room temperature for 30 min.
2. Heat the butter in a large skillet over medium-

high heat. Add the lamb chops and cook for 6 min, then season with salt and pepper.

3. Turn the chops and cook for another 6 min or until cooked to the desired level.

4. Let the lamb chops rest for 5 min before serving.

5. Meanwhile, toss the asparagus with olive oil, salt, and pepper then spread on a baking sheet.

6. Broil for 6 to 8 min until charred, shaking occasionally. Serve hot with the lamb chops.

Nutrition: Calories 685 Fat 52 g Net Carb 3 g Total Carbs: 6 g Fiber: 3 g Protein 50.5 g

WEEK 3

DAY 1

BREAKFAST

262. GRILLED HAWAIIAN BOWL

Prep Time:10 min   **Cooking Time**: 0 min   **Servings** 1

Ingredients

- 2 slices (1/4-inch-thick) grilled fresh pineapple
- 2/3 cup cooked brown rice
- 1/4 cup thinly sliced grilled red onion

Honey-Soy Sauce:
- 1 1/2 tsp. rice vinegar
- 1 tbsp. lower-sodium soy sauce
- 1 tsp. canola oil

- 1/3 cup chopped red bell pepper
- 3 ounces grilled pork tenderloin
- 1/2 cup grilled sliced zucchini

- 1 tsp. honey
- 1/8 tsp. crushed red pepper

Directions:

1. Pineapple-cooked brown rice, red onion, red bell pepper, grilled pork and zucchini.

2. Combine the soy sauce, vinegar, sugar, canola oil, and crushed red pepper in a small bowl and blend well with a whisk. Spread over a mug.

Nutrition: Calories 393 Satfat 1.4g Fat 10.8g Polyfat 2g Monofat 4.8g Carbohydrate 56g Protein 22g Cholesterol 45mg Fiber 6g Sodium 588mg Iron 3mg Sugars 22g Calcium 41mg Est. added sugars 6g

LUNCH

263. PORK WRAPS

Prep Time:15 min   **Cooking Time**: 5 min   **Servings** 4

Ingredients

- 1 tbsp. minced peeled fresh ginger
- 1 tbsp. dark sesame oil
- 1 cup matchstick-cut carrot
- 5 garlic cloves, minced
- 1 cup (1-inch) pieces green onions
- 2 (3.5-ounce) packages sliced fresh shiitake mushrooms
- 1/8 tsp. kosher salt

- 4 cups thinly sliced napa cabbage
- 12 ounces boneless pork shoulder, trimmed and very thinly sliced
- 1 tsp. sugar
- Cooking spray
- 1 tbsp. hoisin sauce
- 1 1/2 tbsp. water
- 8 (6.5-inch) whole-wheat tortilla

Directions:

1. Over medium heat, heat a large skillet. In a pan, add oil; swirl to coat. Add the ginger and garlic; cook for 30 seconds, continuously stirring. Raise the heat to medium-high heat. Add the mushrooms and carrot; cook for 2 min, stirring frequently. Add the cabbage and onions; cook for 1 to 2 min or until the cabbage wilts. Spoon the mixture of cabbage into a large bowl; stir in the salt.

2. With paper towels, wipe the pan clean. Bring the pan back to medium-high heat. Mix the sugar and pork together, tossing well to coat. Cover pan with spray for cooking. Add the mixture of pork to the pan; cook for 3 min or until the pork is browned and done, stirring occasionally. Add 1 1/2 tbsp. of

water to the pan carefully, scraping the pan to loosen the browned pieces. Incorporate the hoisin sauce. Apply the mixture of cabbage to the pan; gently toss to blend. Spoon each tortilla with about 2/3 of a cup of pork mixture, roll-up.

Nutrition: Calories 391 Satfat 4.6g Fat 14.1g Polyfat 3g Monofat 6.2g Carbohydrate 40g Protein 25g Cholesterol 57mg Fiber 20g Sodium 676mg Iron 3mg Sugars 8g Calcium 231mg Est. added sugars 2g

DINNER

264. STRAWBERRY-CHICKEN SALAD WITH PECANS

Prep Time: 15 min   **Cooking Time:** 5 min   **Servings** 2

Ingredients

- 1 tbsp. white balsamic vinegar
- 4 tsp. extra-virgin olive oil, divided
- 1/2 tsp. chopped fresh thyme
- 1 tsp. honey
- 1/4 tsp. kosher salt, divided
- 3/8 tsp. freshly ground black pepper, divided
- 2 cups halved strawberries, divided
- 3/8 tsp. freshly ground black pepper, divided
- 1/4 tsp. smoked paprika
- 2 (4-ounce) skinless, boneless chicken breast cutlets
- Cooking spray
- 1/4 cup thinly sliced red onion
- 4 cups fresh baby spinach
- 1 ounce reduced-fat feta cheese, crumbled (about 1/4 cup)
- 3 tbsp. chopped pecans, toasted

Directions:

1. In a medium cup, combine vinegar, one tbsp. oil, thyme, honey, 1/4 tsp. pepper, and 1/8 tsp. salt; blend with a whisk. Attach 1 cup of strawberries and toss to cover. Let it stand for 10 min at room temperature.
2. Over medium-high heat, heat a medium skillet. Brush the chicken with one tsp. of oil remaining; sprinkle with the remaining 1/8 tsp. of pepper, salt, and paprika evenly. Cover pan with spray for cooking. Add the chicken to the pan; cook on each side or until cooked, 2 to 3 min. Take the chicken out of the pan; leave to stand for 5 min. Cut into slices across the grain.
3. Divide the spinach into two plates, the remaining 1 cup of strawberries, and the onion. Using chicken slices as well as a strawberry-balsamic mixture to top evenly. Top with 1 1/2 tbsp. of pecans and two tbsp. of cheese for each serving.

Nutrition: Calories 399 Satfat 3.9g Fat 22.2g Polyfat 4g Monofat 11.7g Carbohydrate 22g Protein 31g Cholesterol 77mg Fiber 6g Sodium 619mg Iron 3mg Sugars 12g Calcium 147mg Est. added sugars 3g

DAY 2

BREAKFAST

265. TOFU AND NOODLE BOWL WITH CARAMELIZED COCONUT

Prep Time : 20 min   **Cooking Time:** 15 min   **Servings** 4

Ingredients

- 1 tsp. grated peeled fresh ginger
- 2 tsp. grated fresh jalapeño pepper
- 1 garlic clove, grated
- 1 (13.5-ounce) can light coconut milk
- 6 ounces dried brown rice noodles (such as Annie Chun's)
- 1 (14-ounce) package extra-firm water-packed tofu, drained and cut into 1/2-inch cubes
- 1/2 cup unsalted vegetable stock
- 1 1/2 cups frozen edamame
- 3/4 tsp. kosher salt
- 1 1/2 tbsp. fresh lime juice
- 1/4 cup chopped unsalted, dry-roasted peanuts
- 6 ounces baby spinach

Directions:

1. Combine a large skillet with the first 4 ingredients; bring to a boil. Tofu is applied to the pan. Cook for 12 min or until the liquid is reduced to about 1/3 cup and begins to turn golden light, stirring regularly.
2. According to package instructions, prepare rice noodles, omitting salt and fat. At the last

min of cooking, add the edamame to the noodles. Set aside 1/2 of a cup of cooking liquid. Drain the noodle mixture; apply cold water to rinse, then drain.

3. Add the mixture of noodles, stock, and 1/2 cup of reserved cooking liquid into the pan; toss to cover. Stir in the juice, salt, and spinach. Remove from the sun. Sprinkle peanuts on them.

Nutrition: Calories 393 Satfat 2.8g Fat 13.6g Polyfat 5g Monofat 3.4g Carbohydrate 52g Protein 18g Cholesterol 0.0mg Fiber 5g Sodium 469mg Iron 5mg Calcium 145mg

LUNCH

266. KOREAN SHRIMP BBQ BOWL

Prep Time :20 min   **Cooking Time:** 15 min   **Servings** 1

Ingredients

- 1 ounce shiitake mushrooms
- 2 cups fresh spinach
- 2/3 cup cooked brown rice
- 1/2 tsp. canola oil
- 1/3 cup shredded cabbage
- 1 fried egg
- 1/3 cup matchstick-cut carrot
- 3 ounces pan-seared large shrimp
- 2 tbsp. chopped green onions

Spicy Aioli:
- 1 1/2 tsp. canola mayonnaise
- 2 tsp. gochujang (Korean chile sauce)
- 1 small garlic clove, minced
- 1/4 tsp. dark sesame oil

Directions:

1. Sauté the mushrooms and spinach in canola oil. Cooked brown rice with a blend of wilted spinach, carrot, cabbage, shrimp, green onions, and egg.

2. Combine the mayonnaise, gochujang, sesame oil, and minced garlic in a small bowl. Drizzle over tub.

Nutrition: Calories 400 Satfat 2.2g Fat 14.3g Polyfat 3.2g Monofat 5.3g Est. added sugars 3g Carbohydrate 43g Protein 27g Cholesterol 311mg Fiber 6g Sodium 595mg Iron 4mg Sugars 7g Calcium 177mg

DINNER

267. STEAK TACOS

Prep. Time - 2 Hours 25 Mins   **Cooking Time** - 25 Mins   **Servings** 6

Ingredients

- 1/4 cup olive oil, divided
- 1 medium red onion, peeled and cut into 1/2-inch-thick slices
- 2 dried chiles de arbol
- 1/4 cup Mexican crema
- 5 garlic cloves, minced
- 1 (1 1/2-pound) flat iron or skirt steak
- 5 tbsp. fresh lime juice
- Cooking spray
- 3/4 tsp. kosher salt
- 3/4 cup Toasted Chile Salsa
- 12 Fresh Corn Tortillas or packaged corn tortillas, warmed

Directions:

1. Over high cook, cook a cast-iron skillet. Add onion; cook, turning once, for 5 min or until charred. Remove from pan; chop and put in a bowl.

2. Over medium heat, heat a small skillet. To the tub, apply two tbsp. of oil. Add garlic and chiles; cook two min, stirring occasionally. In a cup, apply the garlic mixture to the onion. Incorporate the juice and remaining oil. Mix half of the onion mixture (including both chiles de árbol) as well as steak in a large zip-top plastic bag; seal. Refrigerate 1 hour. Reserve the remaining mixture of onions. Remove

the steak from the fridge; leave to stand for 1 hour at room temperature. Preheat the grill to a medium-high temperature.

3. Remove steak from marinade; discard marinade. Wipe off the steak with any remaining onion and garlic. Sprinkle salt with the steak. Place the steak on a spray-coated grill rack; grill over medium-high heat for 8 min or until desired, turning once. Set aside from the grill; leave to stand for 15 min.

4. Cut the steak into very thin slices around the grain. To the reserved onion mixture, add the steak and accumulated juices, toss. Put two tortillas on six

plates each. Top each tortilla with the 1 1/2 ounces of steak; divide onion mixture among tacos. Place one tbsp. of Toasted Chile Salsa and one tsp. of cream each on top.

Nutrition: Calories 395 Satfat 4.6g Fat 18.3g Polyfat 1.2g Monofat 7.7g Carbohydrate 30g Protein 27g Cholesterol 81mg Fiber 3g Sodium 574mg Iron 6mg Sugars 2g Calcium 71mg Est. added sugars 0g

DAY 3

BREAKFAST

268.   STEAK AND ROASTED SWEET POTATO BOWL

Prep Time :10 min   **Cooking Time:** 0 min   **Servings** 1

Ingredients

- 1 tbsp. salsa verde
- 1/2 cup cooked brown rice
- 2 tbsp. thinly sliced peeled avocado
- 1/3 cup black beans
- 1 1/2 ounces grilled flank steak
- 1/2 cup cubed roasted sweet potato
- 2 tbsp. fresh cilantro
- 1 tbsp. roasted pumpkin seed kernels
- 1 tsp. olive oil
- Honey-Chipotle-Lime Sauce:
- 1/2 tsp. honey
- 1 tsp. adobo sauce
- 1 tsp. fresh lime juice

Directions:

1. Mix the cooked brown rice along with the salsa verde. Black beans, avocado, sweet potato, steak, kernels of pumpkin seeds, and cilantro on top.

2. Combine the olive oil, adobo sauce, sugar, and lime juice in a small bowl and whisk in a small bowl. Sprinkle over the bowl of steak.

Nutrition: Calories 398 Satfat 2.3g Fat 12.4g Polyfat 1.2g Monofat 6.4g Carbohydrate 52g Protein 21g Cholesterol 32mg Fiber 10g Sodium 438mg Iron 3mg Sugars 7g Calcium 73mg Est. added sugars 3g

LUNCH

269.   CHICKEN AND BLACK BEAN ENCHILADAS

Prep. Time - 1 Hour 45 Mins   **Cooking Time** - 23 Mins   **Servings** 8

Ingredients

- Cooking spray
- 1 1/2 cups chopped onion
- 1 tbsp. canola oil
- 5 garlic cloves, minced
- 1 cup chopped poblano chile
- 1 tsp. ground cumin
- 2 tsp. chili powder
- 1 cup unsalted chicken stock
- 1/2 tsp. dried oregano
- 2 (8-ounce) cans unsalted tomato sauce
- 1 tbsp. pureed canned chipotle chiles in adobo sauce
- 1 (15.5-ounce) can unsalted black beans, rinsed and drained
- 3 cups shredded cooked skinless chicken breast
- 4 ounces shredded part-skim mozzarella cheese (about 1 cup)
- 4 ounces shredded reduced-fat cheddar cheese (about 1 cup)
- 1 cup prepared salsa
- 16 (6-inch) corn tortillas
- Fresh cilantro leaves (optional)
- 1/2 cup reduced-fat sour cream

Directions:

1. Preheat the oven to 350 degrees. Using cooking spray to cover a 13 x 9-inch baking dish.
2. Heat oil over medium heat in a large skillet. Add the onion, poblano, and garlic and sauté for 4 min or until the poblano and onion are tender. Stir in chili powder, cumin and oregano. Add stock, chipotle, and tomato sauce and simmer; cook for 5 min or until slightly thickened.
3. In a medium bowl, combine the chicken and the black beans; add half the sauce mixture. Combine the cheeses in a bowl; blend the chicken mixture with 1/2 cup cheese mixture. To combine, toss.

4. Put eight tortillas on a microwave-safe plate; cover with a paper towel that is slightly damp. Microwave for 45 seconds at HIGH or until warm. Place the tortilla on a flat work surface, operating with one tortilla at a time; spoon 1/4 cup chicken mixture on one end of the tortilla. Roll up, style jelly-roll. Repeat the process for leftover tortillas when the first batch is used up, heating up the second batch of tortillas. Arrange the enchiladas in the prepared bowl, seam side down. Sprinkle with the remaining the cheese mixture; pour the remaining sauce over the enchiladas. Bake for thirteen min or until the sauce is bubbly and the cheese is melted and golden brown, uncovered, at 350 °. When needed, serve enchiladas with salsa, sour cream, and cilantro.

Nutrition: Calories 406 Satfat 5.4g Fat 13.1g Polyfat 1.8g Monofat 2.9g Carbohydrate 42g Protein 32g Est. added sugars 1g Cholesterol 70mg Fiber 8g Sodium 531mg Iron 3mg Sugars 7g Calcium 435mg

DINNER
270. ROASTED SALMON WITH WINE COUSCOUS
Prep. Time: 45 Mins **Cooking Time** 15 Mins **Servings** 4

- 2 tbsp. chopped fresh chives
- 2 tbsp. 2% reduced-fat Greek yogurt
- 4 tsp. lemon juice, divided
- 2 tbsp. olive oil, divided
- 1 1/8 tsp. kosher salt, divided
- 4 (6-ounce) salmon fillets
- 2 cups finely chopped carrots
- 1/2 tsp. black pepper, divided
- 2 tsp. minced garlic
- 1/4 cup minced shallots
- 1 cup hot cooked couscous
- 1/3 cup dry white wine

Directions:
1. Preheat the oven to 450 degrees. Combine the yogurt, chives, two tsp. of oil, and one tbsp. of juice and whisk together. Sprinkle 1/2 tsp. salt and 1/4 tsp. pepper over the fish. Rub with a mixture of 2 tsp. yogurt. Over high heat, heat an ovenproof skillet. To the pan, add one tsp. of oil. Add fish, side down on the skin; cook for 2 min. Turn to the oven. Bake for 5 min at 450 °. Turn the fish over; cook for 1 min or until ready.

2. Over medium-high prepare, prepare a skillet. To the tub, apply the remaining one tbsp. of oil. Add the carrots, shallots, and garlic; cook, occasionally stirring, for 4 min. Apply the remaining one tsp. of lemon juice, the remaining 5/8 of a tsp. of salt, 1/4 of a tsp. of pepper and wine. 30 seconds to cook. Stir in couscous; toss. Serve the fish with a combination of couscous and yogurt.

Nutrition: Calories 404 Satfat 2.7g Fat 17.9g Polyfat 5.1g Monofat 8.5g Est. added sugars 0g Carbohydrate 19g Protein 37g Cholesterol 94mg Fiber 3g Sodium 667mg Iron 2mg Sugars 4g Calcium 59mg

DAY 4

BREAKFAST
271. VEGETARIAN TORTILLA SOUP
Prep. Time: 5 Min **Cooking Time**: 25 Min **Servings**: 4
Ingredients

- 2 tsp. olive oil
- 2 cloves garlic, minced
- 1 onion, diced
- 1 tsp. cumin
- 2 tsp. paprika
- 3/4 tsp. chili powder
- 3/4 tsp. coriander
- 14 oz. crushed tomatoes
- 1/8 tsp. cayenne pepper
- 14 oz. canned hominy, rinsed and drained
- 4 cups vegetable broth
- 2 limes
- 1 cup corn (frozen or canned)
- 1/4 cup cilantro
- 14 oz. canned black beans, rinsed and drained
- 2 corn tortillas
- 2 oz queso fresco
- 2 radishes, sliced into super thin rounds

Directions:
1. To 400 degrees, preheat the oven. Heat the olive oil over high-medium heat. Add the onion and cook for approximately 4-5 min. Garlic is added and cooked for 30 seconds. Spices are added and cook for 30 seconds.

2. Add the broth and the crushed tomatoes. Together, stir. You may want to use an immersion blender at this stage to mix the tomatoes and broth if you want a smoother soup.

3. Add the black beans and hominy. Boil for 20 min.

4. Break your tortillas into tiny strips. Use cooking spray to sprinkle and put on a baking sheet or foil. Bake until crispy for 6-8 min.

5. Crunchy strips of tortillas, cheese, cilantro, radishes, and lime juice.

Nutrition: Calories 312, Monounsaturated Fat 0g, Cholesterol 10mg, Saturated Fat 2g, Total Carbohydrate 55g, Polyunsaturated Fat 0g, Sodium 1786mg, Dietary Fiber 15g, Sugars 10g, Total Fat 8g, Protein 13g.

LUNCH
272. PARMESAN BROCCOLI PASTA

Prep. Time: 5 Min   **Cooking Time:** 20 Min   **Servings:** 4

Ingredients
- 2 tsp. olive oil
- 8 oz. high fiber pasta
- 4 cloves garlic, minced
- 1 cup skim milk (add more if needed)
- 2 cups vegetable broth
- 1/2 cup Parmesan cheese
- 3 cups broccoli florets
- Salt and pepper

Directions:
1. Heat the olive oil over high-medium heat. Add garlic and cook until fragrant, for 1-2 min. Pasta, broth, and milk should be added together. Carry to a boil and then to a simmer; turn down. Cook, sometimes stirring, for 18-20 min. After 8 min, add the broccoli. To make a creamy sauce, cook until the pasta is completely cooked, and the fluid is absorbed. Add more milk or vegetable broth if needed.
2. Stir in the cheese with Parmesan. Using salt and plenty of black pepper to season.

Nutrition: Calories 300, Saturated Fat 3g, Polyunsaturated Fat 0g, Total Carbohydrate 52g, Monounsaturated Fat 0g, Total Fat 12g, Sodium 751mg, Sugars 7g, Dietary Fiber 8g, Cholesterol 11mg, Protein 15g.

DINNER
273. CHICKEN PARMESAN ZUCCHINI BOATS

Prep. Time: 15 Min   **Cooking Time:** 35 Min   **Servings:** 5

Ingredients
- 5 zucchini
- 2 garlic clove, minced
- 1 cup part skim shredded mozzarella cheese
- 1/2 cup onion, diced
- 2 tsp olive oil
- 1/4 cup basil, chopped
- 1 lb 99% lean ground chicken (or chopped chicken breast)
- 1/2 tsp oregano
- 14 oz canned diced Italian tomatoes, drained

Directions:
1. To 400, preheat the oven.
2. To build a ship, slice the zucchini and scoop out the centers with a spatula. Finely chop the scooped-out zucchini.
3. Over medium flame heat the olive oil. Add the chicken and onion from the ground. Cook for 6-8 min until it is not pink anymore.
4. Garlic, chopped zucchini, diced tomatoes, basil, and oregano are added to the altogether. Cook until fragrant for 2-3 min.
5. Place it in a baking dish with the zucchini. Fill the mixture with chicken. With shredded cheese on top.
6. Using foil to cover and bake for 25 min. Then remove the foil and bake for another 10 min.

Nutrition Calories 267, Monounsaturated Fat 1g, Saturated Fat 4g, Sodium 359mg, Polyunsaturated Fat 0g, Dietary Fiber 4gm, Total Fat 11g, Total Carbohydrate 16g, Sugars 11g, Cholesterol 76mg, Protein 27g.

DAY 5

BREAKFAST
274. STEAK AND ROASTED SWEET POTATO BOWL

Prep. Time: 15 Min   **Cooking Time:** 0 Min   **Servings:** 1

Ingredients
- 1 tbsp. salsa verde
- 1/2 cup cooked brown rice
- 2 tbsp. thinly sliced peeled avocado
- 1/3 cup black beans

- 1 1/2 ounces grilled flank steak
- 1/2 cup cubed roasted sweet potato
- 2 tbsp. fresh cilantro
- 1 tbsp. roasted pumpkin seed kernels
- 1 tsp. olive oil

- Honey-Chipotle-Lime Sauce:
- 1/2 tsp. honey
- 1 tsp. adobo sauce
- 1 tsp. fresh lime juice

Directions:

1. Mix the cooked brown rice along with the salsa verde. Black beans, avocado, sweet potato, steak, kernels of pumpkin seeds, and cilantro on top.

2. Combine the olive oil, adobo sauce, sugar, and lime juice in a small bowl and whisk in a small bowl. Sprinkle over the bowl of steak.

Nutrition: Calories 398 Satfat 2.3g Fat 12.4g Polyfat 1.2g Monofat 6.4g Carbohydrate 52g Protein 21g Cholesterol 32mg Fiber 10g Sodium 438mg Iron 3mg Sugars 7g Calcium 73mg Est. added sugars 3g

LUNCH

275.   SPICY CHICKEN WINGS

Prep Time: 20 min   **Cooking Time:** 30 min   **Servings:** 4

Ingredients:

- 2 lb. Chicken Wings
- 1 tsp. Cajun Spice
- 2 tsp. Smoked Paprika

- ½ tsp. Turmeric
- Salt - Dash
- 2 tbsp. Baking Powder

- Pepper - Dash.

Directions:

1. When you first begin the Ketogenic Diet, you may find that you won't be eating the traditional foods that may have made up a majority of your diet in the past. While this is a good thing for your health, you may feel you are missing out! The good news is that there are delicious alternatives that aren't lacking in flavor!

2. To start this recipe, you'll want to prep the stove to 400°F. As this heat up, you will want to take some time to dry your chicken wings with a paper towel. This will help remove any excess moisture and get you some nice, crispy wings!

3. When you are all set, take out a mixing bowl and place all of the seasonings along with the baking powder. If you feel like it, you can adjust the seasoning levels however you would like.

4. Once these are set, go ahead and throw the chicken wings in and coat evenly.

5. If you have one, you'll want to place the wings on a wire rack that is placed over your baking tray. If not, you can just lay them across the baking sheet.

6. Now that your chicken wings are set, you are going to pop them into the stove for 30 min.

7. By the end of this time, the tops of the wings should be crispy. If they are, take them out from the oven and flip them so that you can bake the other side.

8. You will want to cook these for an additional 30 min.

9. Finally, take the tray from the oven and allow it to cool slightly before serving up your spiced keto wings. For additional flavor, serve with any of your favorite, keto-friendly dipping sauce.

Nutrition: Calories 299 kcal Fats: 7 g Carbs: 1 g Proteins: 60 g.

DINNER

276.   LEMONY ROASTED SALMON WITH WHITE WINE COUSCOUS

Prep. Time: 25 Mins   **Cooking Time:** 15 Mins   **Servings:** 4

Ingredients

- 2 tbsp. chopped fresh chives
- 2 tbsp. 2% reduced-fat Greek yogurt
- 4 tsp. lemon juice, divided
- 2 tbsp. olive oil, divided

- 1 1/8 tsp. kosher salt, divided
- 4 (6-ounce) salmon fillets
- 2 cups finely chopped carrots
- 1/2 tsp. black pepper, divided

- 2 tsp. minced garlic
- 1/4 cup minced shallots
- 1 cup hot cooked couscous
- 1/3 cup dry white wine

Directions:

1. Preheat the oven to 450 degrees. Combine the yogurt, chives, two tsp. of oil, and one tbsp. of juice and whisk together. Sprinkle 1/2 tsp. salt and 1/4 tsp. pepper over the fish. Rub with a mixture

of 2 tsp. yogurt. Over high heat, heat an ovenproof skillet. To the pan, add one tsp. of oil. Add fish, side down on the skin; cook for 2 min. Turn to the oven. Bake for 5 min. at 450 °. Turn the fish over; cook for 1 min. or until ready.

2. Over medium-high prepare, prepare a skillet. To the tub, apply the remaining one tbsp. of oil. Add the carrots, shallots, and garlic; cook, occasionally stirring, for 4 min. Apply the remaining one tsp. of lemon juice, the remaining 5/8 of a tsp. of salt, 1/4 of a tsp. of pepper and wine. 30 seconds to cook. Stir in couscous; toss. Serve the fish with a combination of couscous and yogurt.

Nutrition: Calories 404 Satfat 2.7g Fat 17.9g Polyfat 5.1g Monofat 8.5g Carbohydrate 19g Protein 37g Cholesterol 94mg Fiber 3g Sodium 667mg Iron 2mg Sugars 4g Calcium 59mg Est. added sugars 0g

DAY 6

BREAKFAST

277.   MEATBALLS AND PEPPERS IN GRAVY

Prep. Time: 20 Min.   **Cooking Time**: 20 Min.   **Servings**: 4

Ingredients

- 1 lb. 95% lean ground beef
- 2 tsp. Italian seasoning
- 1/4 cup onion, minced
- 12 oz. nonfat evaporated milk
- 1/2 tsp. pepper
- 2 tsp. olive oil
- 1/2 tsp. salt
- 1 red bell pepper, chopped
- 1 cup mushrooms, sliced
- 1 yellow bell pepper, chopped
- 3 garlic cloves, minced
- 1 summer squash, chopped
- 1.25 tbsp. whole wheat flour (substitute 1 tsp. cornstarch or arrowroot for low carb/Paleo/GF)

Directions:

1. Mix the onion, beef, salt, Italian seasoning, and pepper together. Consider adding 1⁄4-1 tsp, if you like heat—likewise, red pepper flakes.

2. Roll this mixture into 20 meatballs with a diameter of about 1 inch. Over medium flame heat the olive oil. Add the meatballs and cook until browned on all sides, for 4-5 min. Turn the heat down and continue to cook for 15 min. until it is cooked. Remove and set aside. Tent with foil to preserve the warmth.

3. Using the skillet to add the tomatoes, mushrooms, squash, and garlic. Cook until just tender, for 4-5 min.

4. Mix 1 tbsp. Of evaporated milk with the flour. Add and stir well into the pan.

5. Add the remaining evaporated milk and cook until the sauce is thick, for around 5-8 min.—season with salt and pepper. To mix everything, add the meatballs to the pan and stir.

Nutrition: Calories 280, Saturated Fat 3g, Polyunsaturated Fat 0g, Monounsaturated Fat 2g, Total Fat 8g, Sodium 472mg, Cholesterol 74mg, Dietary Fiber 2g, Sugars 13g, Total Carbohydrate 19g, Protein 33g.

LUNCH

278.   HAM QUICHE WITH CHEESE

Prep Time: 10 min   **Cooking Time**: 30 min   **Servings**: 6

Ingredients:

- 8 eggs
- 1 cup Zucchini
- ½ cup Shredded heavy Cream
- 1 cup Ham, Diced
- 1 tsp. Mustard
- Salt – Dash.

Directions:

1. For this recipe, you can start off by prepping your stove to 375°F and getting out a pie plate for your quiche. Next, it is time to prep the zucchini. First, you will want to go ahead and shred it into small pieces. Once this is complete, take a paper towel and gently squeeze out the excess moisture. This will help avoid a soggy quiche.

2. When the step from above is complete, you will want to place the zucchini into your pie plate along with the cooked ham pieces and your cheese.

3. Once these items are in place, you will want to whisk the seasonings, cream, and eggs together before pouring it over the top.

4. Now that your quiche is set, you are going to pop the dish into your stove for about 40min.

5. By the end of this time, the egg should be cooked through, and you will be able to insert a knife into the center and have it come out clean.

6. If the quiche is cooked to your liking, take the dish from the oven and allow it to chill slightly before slicing and serving.

Nutrition: Calories 211 kcal Fats: 25 g Carbs: 2 g Proteins: 20 g.

DINNER

279. TANGY SHRIMP

Prep Time: 15 min   **Cooking Time:** 15 min   **Servings:** 2

Ingredients:

- 3 cloves Garlic
- ¼ cup Olive oil
- ½ lb. Jumbo shrimp
- 1 Lemon
- Cayenne pepper, to taste.

Directions:

1. Sauté the garlic and cayenne with the olive oil.
2. Peel and devein the shrimp.
3. Cook within 2 to 3 min. per side.
4. Put pepper, salt, and lemon wedges.
5. Use the rest of the garlic oil for a dipping sauce. Serve.

Nutrition: Calories: 335 kcal Carbs: 3 g Protein: 23 g Fats: 27 g.

DAY 7

BREAKFAST

280. CRUNCH BOWL WITH SALMON

Prep Time: 15 min   **Cooking Time:** 0 min   **Servings** 1

Ingredients

- 2 tbsp. matchstick-cut carrot
- 2/3 cup cooked quinoa
- 1 tsp. chopped dry-roasted peanuts
- 2 tbsp. steamed edamame
- 2 tbsp. chopped red bell pepper
- 3 ounces broiled salmon

- 1/4 cup shredded red cabbage

Sesame-Peanut Sauce:

- 1 tsp. lower-sodium soy sauce
- 1/2 tsp. fresh lime juice
- 1 tsp. creamy peanut butter
- 1/2 tsp. dark sesame oil
- 1/2 tsp. rice vinegar

Directions:

1. Top-cooked carrot quinoa, red bell pepper, edamame, salmon, and cabbage. Sprinkle peanuts on them.
2. Combine the peanut butter, soy sauce, vinegar, sesame oil, and lime juice in a small cup, stirring well. Spread over a mug.

Nutrition: Calories 397 Satfat 1.9g Fat 15.3g Polyfat 3.3g Monofat 4.3g Carbohydrate 34g Protein 31g Cholesterol 54mg Fiber 6g Sodium 302mg Iron 3mg Sugars 4g Calcium 59mg Est. Added Sugars 0g

LUNCH

281. CARNITAS TACOS WITH RED ONION

Prep Time: 1 Hours 30 Mins   **Cooking Time:** 25 Mins   **Servings** 6

Ingredients

- 1/2 tsp. grated orange rind
- 7 unpeeled garlic cloves
- 4 tsp. achiote paste
- 3 tbsp. fresh orange juice
- 1 3/4 tsp. kosher salt, divided
- 2 tbsp. plus 2 tsp. canola oil, divided
- 1 cup thinly sliced red onion (half-moons)

- 1 (1 1/2-pound) boneless pork shoulder, trimmed
- 1/4 cup cider vinegar
- 1/2 cup water
- 12 Fresh Corn Tortillas or packaged corn tortillas, warmed
- 2 tsp. light agave nectar or granulated sugar
- 3/4 cup Tomatillo Salsa

Directions:

1. Preheat the oven to 250 degrees.
2. Over medium heat, heat a large cast-iron skillet. Add garlic to the pan; cook 8 min. or until the skin is well charred, occasionally turning. Remove the cloves from the pan; cool and discard the skins for 5 min. In a mini chopper, combine the garlic, rind, juice, achiote paste, and two tsp. of oil; process until smooth.

3. Sprinkle the pork with one tsp. of salt. Brush the mixture of achiote evenly over the pork. In a medium Dutch oven or ovenproof saucepan, place the pork; cover and cook for 6 hours at 250 °. Take it out of the oven, and let stand for 30 min.

4. Place the onion in a medium bowl while the pork is cooking. In a saucepan over medium-high heat, mix 1/2 cup water, vinegar, agave, and the remaining 3/4 tsp. salt; bring to a boil, stirring until the salt dissolves. Pour a mixture of vinegar over the onion; stir. Cover the plastic wrap bowl; cool to room temperature, rearranging to hold onion submerged as needed. Chill out for 1 hour, at least.

5. Put pork on a cutting board; shred with two forks. Discard any fat.

6. Over medium-high prepare, heat a large cast-iron skillet. In the pan, add two tbsp. of oil; swirl to coat. In an even layer, add 1 cup of shredded pork to the pan; cook for 3 min. or until a crust forms, turning once. Place the crispy pork on a plate. Repeat procedure with shredded pork remaining.

7. Place two warm tortillas on each of 6 plates. Add 1 1/2 ounces of crisped pork, one tbsp. of Tomatillo Salsa, and one tbsp. of pickled red onion to each tortilla.

Nutrition: Calories 390 Satfat 3.3g Fat 16.1g Polyfat 2.8g Monofat 7.7g Carbohydrate 35g Protein 27g Cholesterol 76mg Fiber 4g Sodium 593mg Iron 4mg Sugars 4g Calcium 88mg Est. added sugars 1g

DINNER

282.   ASPARAGUS, HERB, AND PEA PASTA

Prep Time: 25 Mins   **Cooking Time**: 15 Mins   **Servings** 4

Ingredients

- 1 large garlic clove, thinly sliced
- 2 thin pancetta slices (about 5/8 ounce)
- 3 ounces 1/3-less-fat cream cheese (about 1/3 cup)
- 2/3 cup unsalted chicken stock
- 8 ounces uncooked pappardelle (wide ribbon pasta)
- 3 tbsp. mascarpone cheese
- 1/2 cup frozen green peas
- 1 1/2 cups (1-inch) asparagus pieces
- 1/4 tsp. freshly ground black pepper
- 1/2 tsp. kosher salt
- 1 tbsp. thinly sliced fresh chives
- 1 tbsp. chopped fresh flat-leaf parsley

Directions:

1. Place the pancetta over medium heat in a large skillet; cook for 6 min. or until the pancetta becomes crisp, stirring occasionally. Add the garlic; cook for 30 seconds, continuously stirring. Stock add; bring to a boil.

2. Lower the heat; simmer for 4 min. Add the cream cheese and mascarpone, stirring until smooth with a whisk. Strain sauce over a large bowl through a fine sieve. Solids to discard.

3. Cook pasta according to package instructions; salt and fat are omitted. For the last 2 min. of cooking, add the asparagus and peas; cook for 2 min. Then, drain. In a cup, apply the pasta mixture, salt, and black pepper to the sauce, toss to combine well. Using parsley and chives to sprinkle.

Nutrition: Calories 388 Satfat 5.8g Fat 12.3g Calcium 118mg Polyfat 1.3g Monofat 3g Carbohydrate 53g Protein 17g Cholesterol 61mg Fiber 7g Sodium 407mg Iron 7mg

WEEK 4

DAY 1

BREAKFAST

283.   VANILLA PROTEIN SMOOTHIE

Prep Time: 5 min.   **Cooking Time**: 0 min   **Servings**: 2

Ingredients

- 1 scoop (20g) vanilla egg white protein powder
- ½ cup heavy cream
- ¼ cup vanilla almond milk
- 4 ice cubes
- 1 tbsp. coconut oil
- 1 tbsp. powdered erythritol
- ½ teaspoon vanilla extract
- ¼ cup whipped cream

Directions:

1. Combine all of the ingredients, except the whipped cream, in a blender.
2. Blend on high speed for 30 to 60 seconds until smooth. Pour into a glass and top with whipped cream.

Nutrition: Calories 540 Fat 46 g Net Carb 7.5 g Total Carbs: 8 g Fiber: 0.5 g Protein 25 g

LUNCH
284. CHEESEBURGER SALAD

Prep Time: 10 min.   **Cooking Time**: 10   **Servings**: 2

Ingredients

- 7 ounces ground beef
- Salt and pepper
- 3 tbsp. mayonnaise
- 1 tbsp. diced pickles
- 1 tsp. mustard
- ½ teaspoon ketchup
- Pinch smoked paprika
- 3 ounces chopped romaine lettuce
- 1/3 cup diced tomatoes
- ¼ cup shredded cheddar cheese

Directions:
1. Brown the ground beef over high heat then season with salt and pepper to taste.
2. Drain the fat from the beef and remove from heat.
3. Combine the mayonnaise, pickles, mustard, ketchup, and paprika in a blender.
4. Blend the mixture until smooth and well combined.
5. Combine the lettuce, tomatoes, and cheddar cheese in a mixing bowl.
6. Toss in the ground beef and the dressing until evenly coated.

Nutrition: Calories 395 Fat 27.5 g Total Carbs: 9 g Fiber: 1 g Protein 27.5 g

DINNER
285. CHICKEN ZOODLE CLARISSA

Prep Time: 10 min.   **Cooking Time**: 25   **Servings**: 2

Ingredients

- 2 (6-ounce) chicken breasts
- 1 tbsp. olive oil
- Salt and pepper
- 2 tbsp. butter
- ¼ cup heavy cream
- ¼ cup grated Parmesan cheese
- 200 grams zucchini

Directions:
1. Heat the oil in a large skillet over medium-high heat.
2. Season the chicken with salt and pepper to taste then add to the skillet. Cook for 6 to 7 min. on each side until cooked through then slice into strips.
3. Reheat the skillet over medium-low heat and add the butter.
4. Stir in the heavy cream and Parmesan cheese then cook until thickened.
5. Spiralize the zucchini then toss it into the sauce mixture with the chicken.
6. Cook until the zucchini is tender, about 2 min., then serve hot.

Nutrition: Calories 595 Fat 40 g Net Carb 3 g Total Carbs: 4 g Fiber: 1 g Protein 55 g

DAY 2

BREAKFAST
286. HAM AND CHEESE WAFFLES

Prep Time: 15 min.   **Cooking Time**: 25   **Servings**: 2

Ingredients

- 4 large eggs, divided
- 2 scoops (40 g) egg white protein powder
- 1 teaspoon baking powder
- 1/3 cup melted butter

½ teaspoon salt   1 ounce diced ham   ¼ cup shredded cheddar cheese

Directions:
1. Separate two of the eggs and set the other two aside.
2. Beat 2 of the egg yolks with the protein powder, baking powder, butter, and salt in a mixing bowl.
3. Fold in the chopped ham and grated cheddar cheese. Whisk the egg whites in a separate bowl with a pinch of salt until stiff peaks form.
4. Fold the beaten egg whites into the egg yolk mixture in two batches.
5. Grease a preheated waffle maker then spoon ¼ cup of the batter into it and close it. Cook until the waffle is golden brown, about 3 to 4 min., then remove.
6. Reheat the waffle iron and repeat with the remaining batter. Meanwhile, heat the oil in a skillet and fry the eggs with salt and pepper.
7. Serve the waffles hot, topped with a fried egg.

Nutrition: Calories 575 Fat 46.5 g Net Carb 5 g Total Carbs: 5 g Fiber: 0 g Protein 35 g

LUNCH

287.   PAN-FRIED PEPPERONI PIZZAS

Prep Time: 10 min   **Cooking Time:** 25   **Servings:** 3

Ingredients
- 6 large eggs
- 6 tbsp. grated Parmesan cheese
- 3 tbsp. psyllium husk powder
- 1 ½ tsp. Italian seasoning
- 3 tbsp. olive oil
- 9 tbsp. low-carb tomato sauce, divided
- 4 ½ ounces shredded mozzarella, divided
- 1 ½ ounces diced pepperoni, divided
- 3 tbsp. fresh chopped basil

Directions:
1. Combine the eggs, Parmesan, and psyllium husk powder with the Italian seasoning and a pinch of salt in a blender.
2. Blend until smooth and well combined, about 30 seconds, then rest for 5 min.
3. Heat 1 tbsp. of oil in a skillet over medium-high heat.
4. Spoon 1/3 of the batter into the skillet and spread in a circle then cook until browned underneath.
5. Flip the pizza crust and cook until browned on the other side. Remove the crust to a foil-lined baking sheet and repeat with the remaining batter.
6. Spoon 3 tbsp. of low-carb tomato sauce over each crust. Top with diced pepperoni and shredded cheese then broil until the cheese is browned.
7. Sprinkle with fresh basil then slice the pizza to serve.

Nutrition: Calories 545 Fat 42 g Net Carb 4.5 g Total Carbs: 12 g Fiber: 7.5 g Protein 32 g

DINNER

288.   CABBAGE AND SAUSAGE SKILLET

Prep Time: 10 min.   **Cooking Time:** 20   **Servings:** 4

Ingredients
- 6 large Italian sausage links
- ½ head green cabbage, sliced
- 2 tbsp. butter
- ¼ cup sour cream
- ¼ cup mayonnaise
- Salt and pepper

Directions:
1. Cook the sausage in a skillet over medium-high heat until evenly browned then slice them.
2. Reheat the skillet over medium-high heat then add the butter. Toss in the cabbage and cook until wilted, about 3 to 4 min.
3. Stir the sliced sausage into the cabbage then stir in the sour cream and mayonnaise.
4. Season with salt and pepper then simmer for 10 min.

Nutrition: Calories 350 Fat 24.5 g Net Carb 10 g Total Carbs: 12 g Fiber: 2 g Protein 22 g

DAY 3

BREAKFAST

289.   JACK SAUSAGE EGG MUFFINS

Prep Time: 10 minutes   **Cooking Time**: 30   **Servings**: 3

Ingredients

- 10 ounces ground breakfast sausage
- ½ cup diced yellow onion
- ¼ teaspoon garlic powder
- Salt and pepper
- 3 large eggs, whisked
- 2 tablespoons heavy cream
- ½ cup shredded pepper jack cheese

Directions:

1. Preheat the oven to 350°F and grease three ramekins with cooking spray. Stir together the ground sausage, diced onion, garlic powder, salt, and pepper in a mixing bowl.
2. Divide the sausage mixture evenly in the ramekins, pressing it into the bottom and sides, leaving the middle open.
3. Whisk together the eggs and heavy cream with salt and pepper. Divide the egg mixture among the sausage cups and top with shredded cheese.
4. Bake for 25 to 30 minutes until the eggs are set and the cheese browned.

Nutrition: Calories 455 Fat 37 g Net Carb 3 g Total Carbs: 3.5 g Fiber: 0.5 g Protein 26 g

LUNCH

290.   BACON BURGER BITES

Prep Time: 10 minutes   **Cooking Time**: 15   **Servings**: 16

Ingredients

- 1 lb ground beef
- 8 slices bacon, halved
- 1 large egg, beaten
- 1/2 cup almond flour
- 1/2 tsp garlic powder
- 6 slices mozzarella cheese
- Pickled Jalapeños (optional)
- Salt and pepper, to taste

Directions:

1. Season the meat with garlic powder, salt, and pepper. Crack the egg on the meat and mix well with the almond flour. Knead with your hands or with a spoon to flavor it entirely and create a consistent mixture.
2. Mold into 16 mini meatballs.
3. Prepare 8 strips of bacon and divide into two, making 16 bacon slices. Wrap one slice around one ball.
4. Crispy fry the bacon in two tablespoons of oil using a nonstick frying pan. Remember to cook all sides of the balls.
5. Transfer to a dish once the meatballs turn golden on every side and the bacon is crispy to your liking.
6. Slice the jalapeno into slivers and the cheese into small squares.
7. Top the hot meatballs with a piece of cheese and a slice of jalapeño. Push a toothpick through the ball to hold the tower together. Let the cheese melt on top of the meatball.
8. Enjoy warm with any dip of your choice!

Nutrition: Calories 173 Fat 14.1 g Net Carb 0.6g Total Carbs: 0.7 g Fiber: 0.1 g Protein 10.4 g

DINNER

291.   CHICKEN ALFREDO WITH BROCCOLI

Prep Time: 10 minutes   **Cooking Time**: 15   **Servings**: 4

Ingredients

- 1 lb boneless chicken breast, cut in slices
- 1/2 cup spinach, cut in slices
- 1 cup broccoli florets
- 4 slices bacon (fried and cut into crisp bacon bits)
- 1 tbsp butter
- 1/2 cup heavy cream
- 1 garlic clove minced
- 2 tbsp onion, chopped
- 1/2 tsp salt
- 1/2 tsp pepper

Directions:

1. Give the broccoli the right tenderness and color by placing them in a bowl and pouring some boiling water in. Leave for 10 minutes.
2. On a hot frying pan, sauté the chicken in melted butter with the garlic and onion for 5 minutes.
3. Gently plop the spinach and broccoli into the pan. Add the bacon and cream as well. Season with salt

and pepper to your liking. Leave for another 5 minutes.

Nutrition: Calories 311ng Fat 19.5 g Net Carb 2.5g Total Carbs: 3.3 g Fiber: 0.8 g Protein 31.1 g

4. Pour in a bowl and serve warm.

DAY 4

BREAKFAST

Prep Time: 10 minutes   **Cooking Time**: 15   **Servings**: 4

Ingredients
- 3 cups broccoli
- 1 large egg
- ¼ cup Parmesan cheese, freshly grated
- 1 ½ cup cheddar cheese, shredded
- 2 tsp almond flour
- ½ tsp garlic powder
- Kosher salt
- Black pepper

Directions:

1. Wash and dry your fresh broccoli bunch. Discard all of the leaves before chopping into chunks. Make sure to chop enough chunks for 3 cups.
2. Transfer the chopped broccoli pieces into a food processor. Continue pulsing until you get rice-size bits. Set the microwave to "cooking." Leave the broccoli rice in the microwave for a minute and a half. Crack the egg in a bowl. Add the garlic, cheddar cheese, and almond flour together with the riced broccoli. Beat with a spoon until combined. Season with a dash of pepper and salt.
3. Pat the mixture into a baking tray covered with waxed paper. Cover all sides of the tray evenly.
4. Sprinkle a generous amount of Parmesan cheese on top. Put in the oven for 10 minutes. The oven should be set at 300°F.
5. Take the tray out of the oven. Top with half a cup of cheddar cheese. Rebake for 5 more minutes to melt the cheese. Once ready, remove from the heat. Allow cooling for around 5 minutes then remove the paper.
6. Cut into rectangular shapes and enjoy!

Nutrition: Calories 258 Fat 18.7 g Net Carb 4.1g Total Carbs:6.2 g Fiber: 2.1 g Protein 17.4 g

LUNCH
292.   SALMON SUSHI ROLLS

Prep Time: 30 minutes   **Cooking Time**: 20   **Servings**: 4

Ingredients
Sushi Fillings:
- 2 eggs
- 120 g fresh salmon (or smoked salmon)
- 100 g avocado (1 small)
- 100 g cucumber (1 small)

Sushi Rice:
- 3 cup cauliflower rice (shredded cauliflower)
- 150 g cream cheese, softened
- 2 tbsp rice vinegar
- 1/2 tsp salt, to taste

- 1/2 tsp So Nourished Erythritol (optional)

Other ingredients:
- 2 sheets Nori
- 2 tbsp white sesame seeds
- 1 tsp black sesame seeds (for decoration, optional)
- Sushi dip (optional)
- 1 tbsp ginger, grated
- 1 tbsp lemon juice
- 2 tbsp coconut aminos

Directions:

Making vinegared sushi rice:

1. Wash and cut the cauliflower into small pieces to prepare the cauliflower rice. You can use a knife or a food processor (better choice) to process until obtaining the rice-like pieces.
2. Place the riced cauliflower in a closed container and cook it in the microwave for three minutes. Allow them to cool down. You can also steam or cook the cauliflower in a frying pan. In a mixing bowl, add rice vinegar, sweetener, and salt. Add cauliflower rice and cream cheese in. Stir

everything well with a wooden spoon until you obtain a homogeneous dough.

Prepare sushi fillings and assemble:

1. Peel off the avocado and cucumber skins. Slice into slivers. Slice the salmon into thin slivers too. Scramble egg with a pinch of salt, fry it in a pan, then cut into thin strips.
2. Prep a sushi roller with transparent plastic on both sides to avoid sticking the mixture onto the roller.
3. Place the sushi mat roller on a flat surface. Lay a rectangular nori sheet on top.
4. Split the rice mixture into 2 parts for the 2 nori sheets. Scoop out one part and spread this mixture uniformly over the nori sheet.
5. Arrange the strips of avocado, salmon, egg, and cucumber on one short edge of the sheet. Make sure that the roller can be reeled in that direction.
6. With extra care, roll the filled side up to the other edge of the sheet. Repeat the procedure with the other sheets and remaining mixture.
7. Ideally, chill in the fridge for half an hour before cutting the roll. If desired, simply slice the roll without refrigerating. Slice all sushi rolls into bite-size pieces. This should make 4 servings.

Nutrition: Calories 310 Fat 24 g Net Carb 5.1g Total Carbs: 9.3 g Fiber: 4.2 g Protein 16.4 g

DINNER
293. BUFFALO CHICKEN WINGS
Prep Time: 10 minutes   **Cooking Time:** 15   **Servings:** 4
Ingredients
- 12 chicken wings (whole wings)
- 4 cloves garlic, peeled
- 2 tbsp coconut flour
- 50 ml hot sauce
- 1 tbsp vinegar
- 1 tbsp pepper
- 1 tbsp paprika
- ½ tbsp celery salt
- 1 pinch Stevia (optional)
- 1 lemon (optional)
- Olive oil for deep frying
- 1 tsp salt
- 1 tsp chili pepper

Directions:
1. Coat the chicken wings with lemon on all sides. Set aside for 3 minutes, then wash and dry thoroughly. For a simpler method, just wash and dry the wings without putting in the lemon. Smash together the paprika, pepper, garlic, salt, hot pepper, hot sauce, and vinegar with a mortar
2. Marinate the chicken wings with the mixed spices. Chill in the fridge for an hour while flipping the wings occasionally. Transfer the wings to a plate and coat with coconut flour all over to cover the entire sides.
3. Pour the oil in a deep fryer set at 375°F.
4. Brown the wings in the oil for around 10-15 minutes.
5. Remove from the heat once the wings turn brown on the sides. Serve on a platter.

Nutrition: Calories 300 Fat 17.8 g Net Carb 3.4 g Total Carbs: 7.1 g Fiber: 3.7 g Protein 28.6 g

DAY 5
BREAKFAST
294. AVOCADO SMOOTHIE WITH COCONUT MILK
Prep Time: 10 minutes   **Cooking Time:** 5   **Servings:** 1
Ingredients
- 1 cup coconut milk, unsweetened
- 1 tsp ginger, fresh and grounded
- 1/2 avocado
- 5 leaves spinach
- 1 tsp lime juice (optional)
- 1 tsp Stevia (optional)
- 1 tsp chia seeds

Directions:
1. Wash your ginger and spinach thoroughly.
2. Peel the ginger and avocado. Slice them into pieces.
3. Using a blender, mix all of the ingredients (except chia seeds and stevia) for a minute to obtain a smooth and uniform mixture. Optionally, pour some water and lime juice into the blender to produce the desired thickness. Include some ice cubes and the sweetener into the mix just to flavor it up. Transfer to a glass and garnish with a teaspoon of chia seeds on top. Serve immediately.

Nutrition: Calories 283 Fat 25.3 g Net Carb 4.5 g Total Carbs: 14.4 g Fiber: 9.9 g Protein 3.2 g

LUNCH
295. SPINACH STUFFED CHICKEN

Prep Time: 10 minutes **Cooking Time:** 20 **Servings:** 2

Ingredients

- 1 chicken breast, boneless and skinless
- 1/2 cup chopped spinach
- 1 tbsp onion, chopped
- 1 tbsp butter
- Oil for frying
- 2 tbsp cream cheese
- 1 tbsp grated mozzarella cheese
- Salt and pepper, to taste

Directions:

1. Melt your butter in a hot frying pan. Sauté the spinach and onion in the butter. Set the stove to medium-high heat and leave the vegetables to cook for about 3 minutes until soft. Mix the cream cheese in the pan. Allow dissolving for around 2 minutes. Stir to combine with the onion and spinach. Set aside. Slice a pocket in the chicken breast, deep enough to be filled. Rub both sides of the chicken with salt and pepper. Season all side, including the inside of the pocket.

2. Jampack the pocket with spinach filling and some shredded cheese. Close the breast and secure with a toothpick. Heat the olive oil in a frying pan over medium heat. Gently place the chicken on the oil and cook for 7-10 minutes with the lid on. Turn the chicken over and let it fry for another 7-10 minutes. Remove from the heat once golden.

3. Cut in the middle to spill the filling. Enjoy while warm.

Nutrition: Calories 291 Fat 13.1 g Net Carb 0.9 g Total Carbs: 1.2 g Fiber: 0.3 g Protein 41.7 g

DINNER
296. LOW-CARB NACHOS

Prep Time: 20 minutes **Cooking Time:** 25 **Servings:** 4

Ingredients

For the chips:
- ½ cup almond flour
- 4 slices cheddar cheese (can also use grated mozzarella cheese)
- 2 tbsp butter, melted
- 2 tbsp cream cheese
- 1 small egg (optional)

- 1 tsp salt
- For topping
- 1/2 lb ground beef
- 1/2 tsp dried oregano
- 1 small tomatoes, chopped
- 1 clove garlic, minced
- 1/2 tsp ground pepper
- 2 bay leaves (optional)

For guacamole
- 1 avocado medium-sized, peeled and chopped
- 1 tbsp fresh cilantro, chopped
- 1 small tomato, chopped
- 1 tbsp onion, chopped

Directions:

1. Preheat oven to 350°F.
2. Mix the almond flour, butter, oregano, cream cheese, oregano, and 1 tsp salt in a bowl. Make sure to mix until the dough looks soft so you can use a rolling pin to flatten the dough.
3. Cut small rectangles to form the crackers and place cheddar cheese on each cracker. Place them on a baking sheet and then in the oven for about 10 minutes or until they look brown. Set aside.

4. In the meantime, add oil to a preheated skillet and add the garlic clove, bay leaves, ground beef, pepper, and salt. Let it cook for 10 minutes and then add 2 chopped tomatoes. Cook for 5 more minutes and remove from heat.
5. For the guacamole, mix the avocado, 1 chopped tomato, cilantro, and onion. Add salt to taste.
6. Serve nacho crackers with meat and sour cream on top along with guacamole and enjoy!

Nutrition: Calories 507 Fat 42.1 g Net Carb 4.9 g Total Carbs: 10.5 g Fiber: 5.6 g Protein 26.1 g

DAY 6

BREAKFAST
297. COCONUT PANCAKES

Prep Time: 10 minutes **Cooking Time:** 10 **Servings:** 2

Ingredients

Main Ingredients:

- 2 tbsp coconut flour
- 2 eggs
- ½ tbsp So Nourished Erythritol or a dash of stevia extract
- ¼ tsp baking powder
- 2 tbsp sour cream
- 2 tbsp melted butter
- ½ tsp vanilla extract

For the topping:

- 50 g strawberries
- 1 tbsp shredded coconut
- 1 tbsp almond slices
- 1 tbsp maple syrup (optional)

Directions:

1. Put the eggs, sour cream, 1 ½ tbsp. of melted butter (you'll need the rest for frying the pancakes), vanilla extract, and mix well.
2. Add the coconut flour, baking powder, erythritol to the mixture and mix again. Let the mixture sit for about 15 minutes. If the mixture is too thick, add a little bit of water (20-30 ml) and mix again until the consistency is right. In a pan on medium heat, add butter in and fry the pancakes in butter. The number of pancakes you make will depend on the size you want. We made 6 pancakes with this recipe.
3. Add the toppings and serve!

Nutrition: Calories 274 Fat 23.39 g Net Carb 4.24 g Total Carbs: 8.04 g Fiber: 3.8 g Protein 8.44 g

LUNCH

298. BROCCOLI AND CHICKEN CASSEROLE

Prep Time: 15 min   **Cooking Time**: 35 min   **Servings**: 6

Ingredients:

- 2 tbsp. butter
- ¼ cup cooked bacon, crumbled
- 2½ cups cheddar cheese, shredded and divided
- 4 oz. cream cheese, softened
- ¼ cup heavy whipping cream
- ½ pack ranch seasoning mix
- ⅔ cup homemade chicken broth
- 1½ cups small broccoli florets
- 2 cups cooked grass-fed chicken breast, shredded.

Directions:

1. Preheat your oven to 350°F.
2. Arrange a rack in the upper portion of the oven.
3. For the chicken mixture: In a large wok, melt the butter over low heat.
4. Add the bacon, 1/2 cup of cheddar cheese, cream cheese, heavy whipping cream, ranch seasoning, and broth, and with a wire whisk, beat until well combined. Cook for about 5 minutes, stirring frequently.
5. Meanwhile, in a microwave-safe dish, place the broccoli and microwave until desired tenderness is achieved.
6. In the wok, add the chicken and broccoli and mix until well combined.
7. Remove from the heat and transfer the mixture into a casserole dish. Top the chicken mixture with the remaining cheddar cheese.
8. Bake for about 25 minutes. Now, set the oven to broiler. Broil the chicken mixture for about 2–3 minutes or until cheese is bubbly.
9. Serve hot.

Nutrition: Calories: 431 Fat: 10.5g Fiber: 9.1g Carbs:4.9 g Protein: 14.1g.

DINNER

299. SALMON AND LEMON RELISH

Prep Time: 10 min   **Cooking Time**: 1 h   **Servings**: 2

Ingredients:

- 2 medium salmon fillets
- Black pepper and salt to taste
- 1 shallot, chopped
- 1 tbsp. lemon juice
- 1 big lemon
- ½ cup olive oil

⚑ 2 tbsp. parsley, finely chopped.

Directions:

1. Grease salmon fillets with olive oil, put salt and pepper, place on a lined baking sheet, standing in the oven at 400 °F, and bake for 1 hour
2. Stir 1 tablespoon lemon juice, salt, and pepper in a bowl and leave aside for 10 minutes.
3. Cut the whole lemon in wedges and then very thinly. Put this in shallots, parsley, ¼ cup olive oil, and stir.
4. Break the salmon into medium pieces and serve with the lemon relish on the side.

Nutrition: Calories: 200 kcal Fat: 10 g Carbs: 5 g Fiber: 1 g Protein: 20 g.

DAY 7

BREAKFAST

300. PIZZA BOWL

Prep Time: 5 minutes   **Cooking Time**: 10   **Servings**: 1

Ingredients

⚑ 1/2 green bell pepper, cut in slices

⚑ 1 oz turkey ham, cut in small squares

⚑ 1 tbsp red onion, cut in slices

⚑ 2 tbsp Rao's Pizza Sauce (or tomato paste)

⚑ 1/2 tbsp olive oil

⚑ 1 oz grated mozzarella cheese

Directions:

1. Preheat a frying pan then pour the oil in. Fry the ham for 3 minutes. Optionally, use any meat of your choice instead of ham. Put aside.
2. Set the bell pepper on the base of a microwave-safe bowl. Layer with the onion, ham and finally, tomato paste. Then, top with mozzarella.
3. Microwave for 3 minutes and let the cheese melt. As an alternative, bake for 10 minutes in the oven preheated at 370°F. Remember to use an oven-safe pan for this.
4. Take out from the microwave (or oven) and enjoy!

Nutrition: Calories 213 Fat 15.9 g Net Carb 5.3 g Total Carbs: 7 g Fiber: 1.7 g Protein 11.7 g

LUNCH

301. CHICKEN CORDON BLEU

Prep Time: 5 minutes   **Cooking Time**: 15   **Servings**: 2

Ingredients

⚑ 1 pc chicken breast, boneless and skinless

⚑ 1 lemon (optional)

⚑ 3 slices bacon

⚑ 1 clove garlic, minced

⚑ 1 slice smoked ham

⚑ 1 slice cheddar cheese

⚑ Lettuce (optional)

⚑ Salt and pepper, to taste

Directions:

1. Spray all the sides of the chicken breast with lemon. Set aside for 3 minutes then wash and dry the chicken thoroughly. If there are no lemons available, simply wash and towel dry.
2. Season the chicken with salt, pepper, and minced garlic. Slice the cheese and ham enough to cover the chicken. Lay the ham and cheese slices on top of each chicken breast. Carefully roll the chicken, tuck the ends inside, and finally hold the pieces together with a toothpick.
3. Prepare 3 strips of bacon and wrap them around the rolled up chicken breast.
4. Set an 8-inch non-stick skillet sprayed with cooking spray over medium-high heat.
5. Sear the chicken in the pan, 5 minutes per side until there are no more pink spots on the chicken. Leave in the pan for an additional 2 minutes before removing the toothpick. Lay the chicken on top of a bed of lettuce and serve.
6. If preferred, make the breadcrumb coating for the chicken. Brush the cooked chicken with beaten egg (1 egg or less) and roll it in 2-3 tbsp of almond flour to coat entirely. Crispy fry for 3 minutes until brown.

Nutrition: Calories 56 Fat 19.3 g Net Carb 1.5 g Total Carbs: 1.7 g Fiber: 0.2 g Protein 42.5 g

DINNER

302. SCALLOPS AND FENNEL SAUCE

Prep Time: 10 min   **Cooking Time**: 10 min   **Servings**: 2

Ingredients:

- 6 scallops
- 1 fennel, trimmed, leaves chopped, and bulbs cut in wedges
- ½ lime Juice
- 1 lime zest
- 1 lime, cut in wedges
- 1 egg yolk
- tbsp. ghee, melted and heated up
- ½ tbsp. olive oil
- Black pepper and salt to taste.

Directions:

1 Season scallops with salt and pepper, put in a bowl and mix with half of the lime juice and half of the zest and toss to coat. In a bowl, mix the egg yolk with some salt and pepper, the rest of the lime juice and the rest of the lime zest and whisk well.

2 Add melted ghee and stir very well. Also, add fennel leaves and stir.

3 Brush fennel wedges with oil, place on heated grill over medium-high heat, cook for 2 minutes, flip and cook for 2 minutes more.

4 Add scallops on the grill, cook for 2 minutes, flip and cook for 2 minutes more. Divide fennel and scallops on plates, drizzle fennel and ghee mix and serve with lime wedges on the side. Enjoy!

Nutrition: Calories: 400 kcal Fat: 24 g Fiber: 4 g Carbs: 12 g Protein: 25 g.

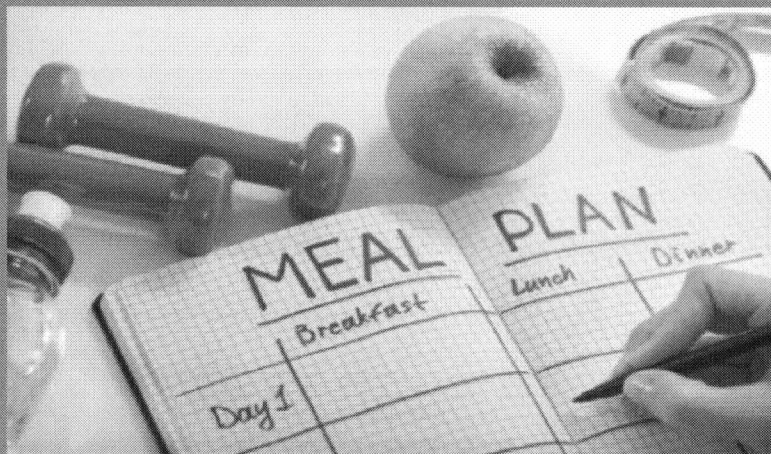

CONCLUSION

The ketogenic diet is a diet that believes that by minimizing carbohydrates while maximizing the good fat in your system and making sure that you are getting the protein you need, that you will be happier and healthier. This book gives you the information to know what this diet is and describe its different types and areas. Most people assume that there is only one way to do it, and while there is one thing that the additional options share, there are four different options that you can choose. Each one has its unique benefits, and you should be familiar with each type to know what would be best for your body, which is why we've outlined them in the book so that you have the best possible information when starting this diet for yourself.

As many people are using this diet to their benefit, learning about food is one of the most significant parts of this, and it becomes easier once you start using this in your daily life. One of the best things you can do is pay attention to the food you are eating and how it affects your body and mind.

The Keto diet has been tried and tested for decades. It originated from a medical background to help patients with epilepsy. Many successful studies align with the knowledge that Keto works. Whether you are trying to diet for a month or a year, both are equally healthy for you. Keto is an adjustment, but it's an adjustment that will continue to benefit you for as long as you can maintain it.

This book has given you all the information you need to do this diet correctly and do it right. It is essential to understand what you are getting into when you embark on this diet, and this book gave you valuable information that you can use to your advantage and avoid the problems that can come with this diet. You want to stay healthy and make sure that your body can do what it needs to do. As with anything, we emphasize that if something seems wrong or unnatural, you will need to see a doctor to make sure you are safe and that your body can handle this diet. Use the knowledge in this book to get amazing recipes and learn directions for excellent meals for yourself.

ACKNOWLEDGMENTS

Thank you for reading this book.

I hope you enjoyed it and found it very valuable and that you are already finding practical ways to start your ketogenic diet and introduce it into your daily life. Doing so is a gift to you and to everyone you will share.

I also hope that you enjoyed the journey through the guide, recipes, and meal plan and that it was helpful for you to hear what the ketogenic diet has to say about the profound change in doing this diet. If you want to read more scientific literature about the science-based diet, follow my books.

If you'd like to get this book in the hands of more people, there are two actions you can take. First and most obvious, please share your copy of the book with someone you think will benefit from reading it or recommending the book to him or her. Second, please take a moment to post a review online or wherever else people are looking for books these days. Your review improves the chances that another person will read the book.

That's a moment of appreciation and salutation, of acknowledging how someone served, even from the bench.

I want to send a special thank you to my friend Elizabeth Roberts, who helped me realize this book. Thank you, Elizabeth, for your precious work!

Good luck on your journey!

And Thank You for Reading this Book!

Eleanor Fields, PhD

Printed in Great Britain
by Amazon